Self-Tracking, Health and Medicine

Sociological Perspectives

Edited by
Deborah Lupton

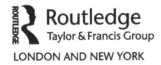

Routledge
Taylor & Francis Group

LONDON AND NEW YORK

First published 2018
by Routledge

2 Park Square, Milton Park, Abingdon, Oxfordshire OX14 4RN
52 Vanderbilt Avenue, New York, NY 10017

Routledge is an imprint of the Taylor & Francis Group, an informa business

First issued in paperback 2019

British Library Cataloguing in Publication Data
A catalogue record for this book is available from the British Library

ISBN 13: 978-1-138-09108-5 (hbk)
ISBN 13: 978-0-367-32186-4 (pbk)

Typeset in Minion Pro
by RefineCatch Limited, Bungay, Suffolk

Publisher's Note
The publisher accepts responsibility for any inconsistencies that may have
arisen during the conversion of this book from journal articles to book chapters,
namely the possible inclusion of journal terminology.

Disclaimer
Every effort has been made to contact copyright holders for their permission to
reprint material in this book. The publishers would be grateful to hear from any
copyright holder who is not here acknowledged and will undertake to rectify
any errors or omissions in future editions of this book.

Self-Tracking, Health and Medicine

Self-tracking practices are part of many health and medical domains. The introduction of digital technologies such as smartphones, tablet computers, apps, social media platforms, dedicated patient support sites and wireless devices for medical monitoring has contributed to the expansion of opportunities for people to engage in self-tracking of their bodies and health and illness states. The contributors to this book cover a range of self-tracking techniques, contexts and geographical locations: fitness tracking using the wearable Fitbit device in the UK; English adolescent girls' use of health and fitness apps; stress and recovery monitoring software and devices in a group of healthy Finns; self-monitoring by young Australian illicit drug users; an Italian diabetes self-care program using an app and web-based software; and 'show-and-tell' videos uploaded to the Quantified Self website about people's experiences of self-tracking. Major themes running across the collection include the emphasis on self-responsibility and self-management on which self-tracking rationales and devices tend to rely; the biopedagogical function of self-tracking (teaching people about how to be both healthy and productive biociti-zens); and the reproduction of social norms and moral meanings concerning health states and embodiment (good health can be achieved through self-tracking, while illness can be avoided or better managed).

This book was originally published as a special issue of the *Health Sociology Review*.

Deborah Lupton is Centenary Research Professor in the News and Media Research Centre, Faculty of Arts and Design at the University of Canberra, Australia. She is the author/co-author of sixteen books, the latest of which are *Digital Sociology* (2015), *The Quantified Self: A Sociology of Self-Tracking* (2016) and *Digital Health: Critical and Cross-Disciplinary Perspectives* (2018).

Contents

Citation Information

The chapters in this book were originally published in the *Health Sociology Review*, volume 26, issue 1 (March 2017). When citing this material, please use the original page numbering for each article, as follows:

For any permission-related enquiries please visit:
http://www.tandfonline.com/page/help/permissions

Notes on Contributors

Annaleise Depper is a PhD student in Health at the University of Bath, UK.

Aristea Fotopoulou is a Research Fellow in Media and Film, University of Sussex, UK.

P. David Howe is a Reader in the Social Anthropology of Sport at Loughborough University, UK.

Deborah Lupton is Centenary Research Professor in the News and Media Research Centre, Faculty of Arts and Design at the University of Canberra, Australia.

Andy Miah is Chair in Science Communication and Future Media at the School of Environment and Life Sciences, University of Salford, UK.

Francesco Miele is based at the Center for Information and Communication Technology, Bruno Kessler Foundation, Italy.

Veera Mustonen is Deputy CEO at the Forum Virium Helsinki, Finland.

Kate O'Riordan is a Reader in Media at the University of Sussex, UK.

Mika Pantzar is based at the Faculty of Social Sciences, Consumer Society Research Centre, University of Helsinki, Finland.

Margaret Pereira is Senior Project Officer at Queensland University of Technology, Australia.

Enrico Maria Piras is a Faculty Member at the Center for Information and Communication Technology, Bruno Kessler Foundation, Italy.

Emma Rich is Senior Lecturer at the Department for Health, University of Bath, UK.

Minna Ruckenstein is Principal Investigator at the Faculty of Social Sciences, Consumer Society Research Centre, University of Helsinki, Finland.

John Scott is Professor at the School of Justice, Faculty of Law, Queensland University of Technology, Australia.

Gavin J. D. Smith is Deputy Head at the School of Sociology, College of Arts and Social Sciences, Australian National University.

Ben Vonthethoff is a researcher at The Regional Australia Institute, Barton, Australia.

Self-tracking, health and medicine

Self-tracking has featured as a central practice in health promotion and healthcare for centuries. People have paid attention to the details of their bodily functions and sensations, their diet, body weight, drug use and exercise habits, as part of attempting to achieve good health or manage illness and disease. Over the past few years, a fascination with self-tracking and its implications for concepts of self, identity, social relations and embodiment has emerged in sociological and other social research. This interest has partly sprung from increasing coverage in the mass media of the potential for new digital technologies to facilitate self-tracking in novel ways. The possibilities for new mobile media and apps to be used to monitor and measure human bodies have also been championed in medical publications (Swan, 2012; Topol, 2015).

The 'quantified self' to describe digital self-tracking has taken on particular cultural resonance. This term first emerged in 2007, when two *Wired* magazine editors, Kevin Kelly and Gary Wolf invented it to describe behaviours that they had observed among colleagues and friends involving the use of digital technologies such as apps and wearable devices to generate detailed personal information about their bodies and elements of their everyday lives. They began organising meetings of people interested in self-tracking and eventually launched a website: The Quantified Self. The quantified self term soon began to appear in the mass media, helped by articles and blog posts penned by Wolf and Kelly for *Wired* and other influential media like *The New York Times*. It began to supplant the older 'lifelogging', which had attracted research interest since the emergence of personal computing, particularly among human–computer interaction (HCI) researchers (Lupton, 2013).

In response to these developments, a body of literature from social researchers has rapidly developed, with at least two books (Lupton, 2016a; Neff & Nafus, 2016) and two edited book collections (Nafus, 2016; Selke, 2016) appearing in 2016. Numerous articles and book chapters about self-tracking have been published since 2012 (for reading lists, see Lupton, 2016b, 2016c). Self-tracking is not always about health and medical issues, but these are key elements. People who engage in reflexive self-monitoring collect information about themselves, and reflect on how this information can be used to improve their lives in some way. These data are often about their bodies and health states: their medical symptoms and medical treatments, sleeping, eating, alcohol and drug use and exercising habits, body weight, blood glucose levels, pulse, moods and stress levels and reproductive and sexual functioning and activities.

While many people engage in self-tracking using non-digital forms of recording their details, such as pen-and-paper or even just relying on their memories (Fox & Duggan, 2013), a vast array of digital technologies have come onto the market that can be used for highly detailed and often automated self-monitoring. There are now over 160,000 health and medical apps on the market, and apps for counting calories, fitness tracking and menstrual cycle tracking are among the most popular in terms of downloads (IMS Institute for Healthcare Informatics, 2015). Wearable devices such as Fitbit, Jawbone Up and Misfit, as well as smartwatches like Apple Watch, have been designed to feature self-tracking sensors and software that can monitor and measure health and bodily movements. Patients with chronic diseases like diabetes, mental health conditions and high blood pressure can use mobile self-monitoring devices and apps to engage in self-care. Patient support platforms such as PatientsLikeMe encourage people to monitor their symptoms and treatments and share these data with others. Exergaming devices like Wii Fit and Kinect Xbox include digital sensors that can monitor and record players' physical activities. Some game apps not obviously directed at self-tracking, such as Pokemon Go, now often include a physical activity monitor as part of the gamification of preventive health.

A particularly intriguing feature of contemporary digitised self-tracking is 'function creep', or the spread of the mentalities, motivations and technologies for self-tracking beyond the personal, domestic or medical sphere into other social domains. I have identified five modes of self-tracking: private, pushed, communal, imposed and exploited (Lupton, 2016a). Many people choose to engage in reflexive self-monitoring voluntarily for their own reasons ('private self-tracking'): because they have decided that they want to lose weight, improve their sleep, get fitter and stronger, feel better, have more energy, feel happier, control their stress levels or be a more productive worker. Self-trackers often find value and comfort in sharing their personal data with other people on social media or specialised physical activity tracking platforms and apps like Strava and providing support to others engaged in similar pursuits ('communal self-tracking'). However, in some instances people are pushed into self-tracking by others. Children may be required to participate in heart-rate monitoring or behaviour monitoring at school using apps or software. Patients with chronic health conditions are sent home by their doctors with the expectation that they will engage in the prescribed self-monitoring program. Employers expect their employees to sign up to workplace 'wellness' programs requiring health and fitness self-tracking. Health and life insurers are beginning to invite clients to upload their medical and exercise data to receive rewards or lower premiums. In other cases, self-tracking is imposed on people: for example, as part of alcohol and other drug monitoring programs. They may have little option but to comply. The data generated from many of these activities are exploited by many different actors and agencies for commercial, managerial, governmental or research purposes.

This special issue of *Health Sociology Review* was designed to highlight recent sociological research and theorising about self-tracking in health and medicine. The seven articles published here cover a range of self-tracking techniques, contexts and geographical locations: fitness tracking using the wearable Fitbit device in the UK (Fotopolou and O'Riordan), English adolescent girls' use of health and fitness apps (Depper and Howe), stress and recovery monitoring software and devices in a group of healthy Finns (Pantzar, Ruckenstein and Mustonen), self-monitoring by young Australian illicit drug users (Pereira and Scott), an Italian diabetes self-care program using an app and web-based software (Piras and Miele) and 'show-and-tell' videos uploaded to the Quantified Self website about people's experiences of self-tracking (Smith and Vonthethoff). Rich and Miah's article takes the form of a review. Focusing on lifestyle apps, they draw attention to the key theoretical perspectives and issues that can be employed to critically analyse these self-tracking artefacts.

The research methods used in the articles are nearly all qualitative. In their studies, Pereira and Scott and Piras and Miele used the classic qualitative method of one-to-one interviews, while Depper and Howe adopted the focus group discussion approach. Smith and Vonthethoff undertook a critical discourse analysis of self-tracking videos and included interviews with two self-trackers to supplement their findings. The authors of two articles experimented with some alternative approaches. Fotopolou and O'Riordan employed a combination of autoethnography, interface analysis of the Fitbit app, device screen and website and qualitative media analysis of news and blogs about Fitbit. Pantzar and colleagues used a combination of analysing the quantitative stress data derived from a self-tracking device plus participants' diary entries and qualitative interviews.

Major themes running across the collection include the emphasis on self-responsibility and self-management on which self-tracking rationales and devices tend to rely, the biopedagogical function of self-tracking (teaching people about how to be both healthy and productive biocitizens) and the reproduction of social norms and moral meanings concerning health states and embodiment (good health can be achieved through self-tracking, while illness can be avoided or better managed). Analysing the ways in which people's bodies and health states are datafied, or rendered into digital data assemblages, and subject to dataveillance, or forms of watching using these data, is addressed in most of the articles.

The authors take up series of theoretical perspectives to analyse the broader implications of health and medical self-tracking. Foucauldian theories of biopower and ethical self-formation are employed in five of the seven articles (Pereira and Scott, Depper and Howe, Fotopolou and O'Riordan, Rich and Miah, Smith and Vonthethoff). Interestingly, Pereira and Scott identify the dominance of moral judgements about the importance of self-management expressed in the young illicit drug users they interviewed. According to these interviewees, 'good' drug-using citizens must make sure that they carefully monitor their drug-taking behaviours to ascribe to guidelines about safe use. Smith and Vonthethoff also take up the work of Beck, Giddens and Lash and their theory of reflexive modernisation to explain the ways in which self-tracking practices are used as part of the project of self-optimisation. They further refer to Bauman's concept of liquid modernity to explain self-tracking as a never-fulfilled quest for self-knowledge and happiness. The satisfactions and comforts of self-tracking, they contend, are ephemeral, because the flows of data generated must constantly be managed and confronted.

Sociomaterial perspectives are adopted in the articles by Pantzar, Ruckenstein and Mustonen and Piras and Miele. Pantzar and colleagues are interested in the intersections between digital self-tracking devices and human actors. They also refer to the work of Lefebvre in focusing attention on the rhythms of life and how these are interembodied. Piras and Miele point to the shared nature of self-tracking as a joint endeavour between patients and doctors where there are often frictions between the different parties' expectations and assumptions of how it should be undertaken. Some of the diabetes patients in Piras and Miele's study sought to challenge or resist the self-tracking practices enjoined upon them by their doctors. They used the self-tracking technology to achieve greater autonomy from surveillance and intervention by doctors. Piras and Miele demonstrate that when doctors attempted to push self-tracking onto patients, patients actively chose how they engage in clinical self-tracking in ways not always expected (or wanted) by their doctors.

Contributions to the existing literature on self-tracking in health and medicine, including the articles in this special issue, have begun to cast light on its sociocultural and political dimensions, including the complex interactions and entanglements between human and non-human actors and between biology and culture. There are many directions that future sociological research can take. Most research thus far, including the articles published in this special issue, has focused on the members of privileged social groups located in the Global North who are tracking their health indicators because they are already conforming to the ideals of the responsibilised, self-managing and entrepreneurial citizen. We know little as yet about how the members of marginalised or stigmatised groups engage in self-tracking, resist it or even re-invent it. How are elderly people, people from minority ethnic or racial groups, people with poor literacy skills or people with disabilities engaging (or not) in self-tracking? How are people living outside the Global North using these technologies?

On the one hand, self-tracking can promote health and wellbeing. On the other hand, it can further contribute to socioeconomic disadvantage and marginalisation. People who do not take up suggestions to self-track their health and fitness by their employers or insurers, for example, may suffer adverse consequences such as being considered as an inadequate employee or paying higher premiums. Research on these populations is ever-more important as people are encouraged or coerced to engage in self-tracking in an increasing number of social domains, and as the personal data generated by self-tracking practices are used in decision-making about funding and service-delivery and thus shape people's life chances.

Personal health and medical data have acquired considerable biovalue in the digital data economy (Lupton, 2016a). They are commonly used for commercial purposes: for instance, developers on-sell them to advertising, medical device and pharmaceutical companies. Data mining companies harvest these data, combining them to create profiles and lists of people identified as having specific medical conditions, and profit from selling these lists to advertising agencies, financial institutions and potential employers (Ebeling, 2016; Pasquale, 2014). Repositories of data about people's sexual activities and preferences, body weight or health conditions can be used to target them for social shaming, exclusion or denial of insurance, credit or employment opportunities (Lupton, 2016a). Sociologists and other social researchers need to identify and draw attention to these uses of personal health and medical data.

Data privacy and security issues also constitute a paramount topic of investigation. The types of personal information about people's bodies that are collected by self-tracking practices can be highly sensitive and revealing of aspects that people may not wish others to know about. Personal data have a 'capacity for betrayal' – they can be 'disloyal' (Nafus, 2014). Medical and health database breaches, including of the data repositories of major hospitals and public health agencies (Gajanayake, Lane, Iannella, & Sahama, 2013; Thilakanathan, Chen, Nepal, Calvo, & Alem, 2014) and health tracking apps (Wicks & Chiauzzi, 2015) frequently occur. Health and medical data are key targets of cybercriminals and hackers, who use the data for fraudulent activities (Ablon, Libicki, & Golay, 2015). Sociologists and other social researchers should continue to investigate these uses of personal health and medical data, both legal and illicit, and highlight the consequences.

The ways in which people incorporate and conceptualise the personal health and medical data they generate from self-tracking as part of their everyday lives and notions of identity and embodiment also require more sustained research. This could include investigations into how people make choices about which kind of information to collect and what practices and devices they use to do so. We have yet to fully understand how people engage with the personal data produced from self-tracking. These data are lively, constantly moving and changing as they are generated and contribute to new forms of data assemblages (Lupton, 2016a). I use the term 'data sense' to encapsulate the complexity of the entanglements between human senses, digital sensors and sense-making in response to these lively data (Lupton, 2016d). How do these data become meaningful – how do they lose meaning? How do people negotiate what their self-tracking devices tell them about their bodies and health, and what their bodily senses reveal to them? What are the sensory and affective dimensions of data sense? In what ways do personal data provide comfort or reassurance – and how do they frustrate or disappoint people? Related to these questions are those concerning data materialisations, or the ways in which digital data are rendered into formats so that people can view them (or in the case of 3D printed objects, even handle them (Lupton, 2015)).

Finally, the ways in which self-tracking technologies and practices are invented, brought onto the market, advocated and incorporated into organisations and institutions also require more attention. What are the decision-making processes by which developers choose to work on self-tracking apps, other software and devices, and what are the tacit assumptions, expectations and norms about bodies and selves underpinning these processes? How are schools and higher education institutions, workplaces, hospitals and other healthcare providers and insurance companies promoting or requiring health and medical self-tracking? What are the intersections between the entrepreneurs and developers working on self-tracking technologies and these institutions and organisations?

The sociology of self-tracking is in its nascent stages. As self-tracking expands further into the domains of social life, and as more people voluntarily take up quantifying themselves or are pushed or coerced to do so, all of these questions, and many more, remain to be answered.

References

Ablon, L., Libicki, M., & Golay, A. (2015). *Markets for cybercrime tools and stolen data*. Santa Monica, CA: RAND Corporation.

Ebeling, M. (2016). *Healthcare and big data: Digital specters and phantom objects*. Houndmills: Palgrave Macmillan.

Fox, S., & Duggan, M. (2013). *Tracking for health*. Retrieved from http://www.pewinternet.org/files/old-media//Files/Reports/2013/PIP_TrackingforHealth20WITH20appendix.pdf

Gajanayake, R., Lane, B., Iannella, R., & Sahama, T. (2013). Accountable-ehealth systems: The next step forward for privacy. *Electronic Journal of Health Informatics, 8*(2), 11. Retrieved from http://www.ejhi.net/ojs/index.php/ejhi/article/view/248

IMS Institute for Healthcare Informatics. (2015). *Patient adoption of mHealth: Use, evidence and remaining barriers to mainstream acceptance*. Parsippany, NJ: IMS Institute for Healthcare Informatics.

Lupton, D. (2013). Understanding the human machine. *IEEE Technology & Society Magazine, 32*(4), 25–30.

Lupton, D. (2015). Fabricated data bodies: Reflections on 3D printed digital body objects in medical and health domains. *Social Theory & Health, 13*(2), 99–115.

Lupton, D. (2016a). *The quantified self: A sociology of self-tracking*. Cambridge: Polity Press.

Lupton, D. (2016b). Critical research on self-tracking: A reading list. *This Sociological Life*. Retrieved from https://simplysociology.wordpress.com/2016/01/12/critical-social-research-on-self-tracking-a-reading-list/

Lupton, D. (2016c). Interesting HCI research on self-tracking: A reading list. *This Sociological Life*. Retrieved from https://simplysociology.wordpress.com/2016/02/15/interesting-hci-research-on-self-tracking-a-reading-list/

Lupton, D. (2016d). Living digital data research program. *This Sociological Life*. Retrieved from https://simplysociology.wordpress.com/2016/02/28/living-digital-data-research-program/

Nafus, D. (2014). Stuck data, dead data, and disloyal data: The stops and starts in making numbers into social practices. *Distinktion: Scandinavian Journal of Social Theory, 15*(2), 208–222.

Nafus, D. (Ed.). (2016). *Quantified: Biosensing technologies in everyday life*. Cambridge, MA: MIT Press.

Neff, G., & Nafus, D. (2016). *Self-tracking*. Cambridge, MA: MIT Press.

Pasquale, F. (2014). The dark market for personal data. *The New York Times*. Retrieved from http://www.nytimes.com/2014/10/17/opinion/the-dark-market-for-personal-data.html

Selke, S. (Ed.). (2016). *Lifelogging: Digital self-tracking and lifelogging – between disruptive technology and cultural transformation*. Wiesbaden: Springer VS.

Swan, M. (2012). Health 2050: The realization of personalized medicine through crowdsourcing, the quantified self, and the participatory biocitizen. *Journal of Personalized Medicine, 2*(3), 93–118.

Thilakanathan, D., Chen, S., Nepal, S., Calvo, R., & Alem, L. (2014). A platform for secure monitoring and sharing of generic health data in the cloud. *Future Generation Computer Systems, 35*, 102–113.

Topol, E. (2015). *The patient will see you now: The future of medicine is in your hands*. New York: Basic Books.

Wicks, P., & Chiauzzi, E. (2015). 'Trust but verify' – five approaches to ensure safe medical apps. *BMC Medicine, 13*(205). Retrieved from http://www.biomedcentral.com/1741-7015/13/205

Deborah Lupton

Health by numbers? Exploring the practice and experience of datafied health

Gavin J. D. Smith and Ben Vonthethoff

ABSTRACT

The widespread availability of portable sensing devices has given rise to growing numbers of people voluntarily self-tracking their daily experiences through the medium of digital data. At the extreme end of this trend is the 'Quantified Self' movement. This collective uses sensor-enabled tech to extensively map aspects of their personal lives, before sharing procedural insights at community 'show and tell' events. A key aim of the group is to better understand imperceptible bodily processes, especially those influencing health states, as they are materialised through the datafied body. Despite the growth in those mobilising digital data for health management, little is known about the subjective meanings that are ascribed to self-monitoring practices. This paper explores how self-trackers conceptualise the data they generate, and how exteriorised bodily interiorities mediate impressions of embodiment. We suggest that the availability of self-tracked data has initiated interesting new relationships between data-subjects and their objectified bodies, dynamics that impact on how bodies are experienced and inhabited. We show how bodily intuition is being outsourced to, if not displaced by, the medium of 'unbodied' data. It is this objectivated facility that is increasingly used to orientate behavioural decisions as they relate to bodily maintenance.

Introduction

> If you want to replace the vagaries of intuition with something more reliable, you first need to gather data. (Wolf, 2010, co-founder of Quantified Self (QS))

Today's world is awash with digital data: data that both structures and represents aspects of human experience, from birth and social relationships to self-identity and death. As people interact with sensor-enabled technologies that are increasingly mobile, networked, and attached to the body – such as smartphones and fitbits – flows of personal data relating to embodied processes and behaviours are created, captured, and circulated. Media devices have afforded new opportunities monitoring, mapping, and visualising everyday events such as eating, running, and expenditure and correlating these with distinct determinants. Although most data are created unconsciously – as people interact with, and through, ambient sensor technologies – there is a growing number of people interested in actively logging their physiologies, movements, moods, and experiences in order to detect previously unseen bodily processes and behavioural habits. This social practice is popularly referred to as 'self-tracking', and it involves the extensive monitoring and measuring of bodily performance and activities via the medium of digital data in order to chart how corporeality relates to external factors.

Underpinning the culture of self-tracking is the idea that data-driven knowledge can provide instruction for those seeking to exercise greater control over their lives. Dalton and Thatcher (2014) contend that the progressive reduction of social life into flows of data requires social scientists to explore how such media 'open up' and 'close off' particular social experiences and practices. As self-tracked digital data are increasingly used to objectify bodily processes in new ways, it becomes imperative to examine how self-tracking transmutes experiences and understandings of embodiment. This is both a conceptual and empirical task. Contemporary healthcare provides an illuminative context in which to analyse this issue: to consider how processes of health provision and consumption are being transformed by practices of self-tracking and the production of digital data.

This paper looks at the QS community, a globally dispersed group of self-trackers who convert selected bodily processes into data as a means to garner insights for the transformation of the embodied self. As a large and diverse contingent deliberately 'prosuming' – that is, producing and consuming – data about their daily habits and biotic states, the QS represents an ideal, if exceptional, sample of people who seek to manage health conditions through the medium of digital data. Notwithstanding the significant growth in those using technologies and digital data for these purposes, little is known about the subjective meanings that are ascribed to self-monitoring practices. In particular, there are limited empirical studies that explore the interrelationship between self-tracking, flows of data, and modes of subjectivity.

We examine how self-trackers in – or on the margins of – the QS community conceptualise and narrate the data they generate, and how the exteriorised data derived from bodily processes subsume their experiences of embodiment. We suggest that the availability of self-tracked data has established interesting new relationships between data-subjects and their objectified bodies, dynamics that have a significant effect on how individuals inhabit their bodies. We point to the way in which the bodily intuition of self-trackers is being outsourced to, if not displaced by, the medium of 'unbodied' data (i.e. from the body, but not of the body). It is this *objectivated* facility (Berger & Luckmann, 1966, pp. 60–61) that is increasingly used as an intuitive device for orientating behavioural decisions as they relate to bodily maintenance.

The reflexive subject and self-tracking practices

Self-tracking repertoires need to be situated within what Beck, Giddens, and Lash (1994) call *reflexive modernisation*, a context in which subjects become increasingly individualised, introspective, and responsible for the project of crafting their own self-identities. Reflexive modernisation is also characterised by a ubiquity of risks which the sovereign state is unable to eradicate, and the consequent need for cosmopolites to manage their own risk loading via the internalisation of expert advice, the exercise of prudent behaviours, and the uptake of available technologies. With these circumstances in mind, it is not difficult to comprehend why some adopt a 'techno-utopian' perspective of self-tracking, perceiving it as a core aspect of preventive medicine (Smarr, 2012; Swan, 2009). While there are indubitable upsides of datafied and devolved health initiatives, these accounts tend to exaggerate the actual capabilities of the technologies, especially by overstating their potential to enable patient empowerment and tangible health benefits. They often fail to acknowledge the 'social, ethical and political implications' of self-monitoring practices and the administration of telecare (Lupton, 2013a, p. 257).

Deborah Lupton (2013a, p. 258), for instance, accentuates the 'digitally engaged patient' notion to describe the way in which lay people are 'encouraged to take an active role in producing and consuming information about health' by using commercial smartphone apps. In this model, patients are expected to assume responsibility for their own health needs via the regimes of personal visibility they enact, representing an archipelago of the medical gaze from the clinic to a more diffuse and plural 'techno-gaze' that permeates any social space mediated through the networked prism of the data sharing device. Lupton (2012, pp. 234–235) argues that these interventions provide individuals with a platform to exteriorise internal bodily dynamics as virtual maps, while simultaneously offering to third-party onlookers 'an unprecedented opportunity to monitor and measure individuals' health-related habits in a variety of milieu'.

The implications of these transformations in contemporary healthcare delivery are not insignificant. For example, Martin French and Gavin Smith (2013) note that encouraging patients to adopt commercially driven tracking devices and infrastructures as a mode of preventive healthcare reflects the neoliberal concern to marketise and outsource the costs and responsibilities of health provisions, while devolving the burden of well-being onto the self-monitoring individual. They point to the implicit assumptions incorporated in these aspirations which tend to presuppose the universal endowment of publics with the resources, skills, and literacy needed to access and operate these technologies. In addition, Gavin Smith (2016) has shown how data-subjects are often neither aware nor in exclusive proprietary possession of the proxy flows of 'disembodied exhaust' that emanate from their bodies. Moreover, Lupton (2015a) has demonstrated that the experience of tracking sexual activity on a number of available smartphone apps is bifurcated as a result of gender codes. For example, those apps designed for female use tend to be framed in terms of the reproductive risks associated with sexual transmitted diseases, while those for men typically focus on enriching sexual stamina and performance. Such platforms are never free of politics and norms, and instead merely reify prevailing gender biases and hierarchies. Significant questions arise regarding how self-tracked data is exploited by different parties for programs of health management (e.g. self-trackers, state agencies, corporations, and insurance actuaries), and how this leakage of information into the bordering 'techno-sphere' impacts on a data-subject's consequent social experiences and life chances (Smith, 2016).

Notwithstanding its potential to render data-subjects susceptible to the gaze of an unknown agency, Nafus and Sherman (2014) suggest that self-tracking represents a form of 'soft resistance' to the monolithic health promotion rhetorics endorsed by governmental agencies and commercial corporations. Such discourses tend to reduce the complexity of health experiences and needs to an idealised – and thus generalised – paradigm. In contrast, personalised notions of 'what is healthy for me?' are particularly common mantras among self-trackers and these individualised self-articulations function to challenge the aggregated definitions of 'healthiness' favoured in medicalised discourses of health, and reflected in the architectures and designs of a number of fitness and self-tracking apps. As such, their concept of 'soft resistance' elucidates how self-trackers conform to broader cultural scripts of maintaining and inhabiting a healthy mind–body, but also shape how this trope is practically achieved at the personal level (Nafus & Sherman, 2014, p. 1785). Yet Lupton (2014b) contends that actual opportunities for soft resistance are limited only to specific modes of voluntary self-tracking. The idea therefore is not necessarily applicable to *involuntary* self-tracking practices such as the measurement of worker productivity by employers or when probationary services subject offenders to mandatory tagging programs. In these examples where the data harvested serves ends and interests above and beyond those of the monitored and objectified subject, possibilities for defiance are severely restricted.

Ruckenstein (2014) found that individuals engaged in self-tracking as a means to make a substantive change in how they organised and performed their personal regimes of health and fitness, especially by being able to retain and analyse better records of bodily physiology and habits over time. She (Ruckenstein, 2014, p. 78) highlights how the virtualised diagram of the body/self visualised through the medium of data intensified self-tracking desires and practices, creating a tangible materialised entity for inspection, measurement, and refinement. Such 'techno-bodied' figures provided self-trackers with opportunities to chart bodily and emotional experiences over time and in relation to specific contexts, catalysts, and events, and to compare these against the social graphs of others. Ruckenstein's focus on motives for self-tracking reveals the nuanced types of social meaning ascribed to experiences of this practice. Inanimate recording units were imbued with symbolic significance and they came to subjectivate the thoughts and actions of those using them. For example, the mere presence of a heart rate monitor in or on the body, and its capacity to connect the bearer to a virtual audience, provided important sources of motivation for the completion of exercise programs.

Research by Hortensius et al. (2012) exposes the *ambiguity* of self-tracking practices, demonstrating how being the object/subject of monitoring can elicit feelings of confidence, certainty, and wholesomeness, while simultaneously generating experiences of anxiety and fragility when the data display unexpected or undesirable results. Yet Nafus and Sherman (2014, p. 1789) argue that self-trackers 'in no way cede authority' to the supposed objectivity of these actants. Nor do they attribute extra validity to their outputs simply because of their quantitative, numeric, and computational attributes. Instead, datafied figures of the body/self act as dialectical mediums through which people *negotiate* meanings.

Our research offers a nuanced conclusion to that of Nafus and Sherman, demonstrating how the datafied figure of the body/self that emerges from self-tracking practices, creates new sensor-based and data-driven and data-driven frameworks for data-subjects to locate bodily intuition and insight. These frameworks function to divert the self-tracker's attention away from the signals and sensations of the embodied sensorium toward a technical sensing apparatus that uses algorithmic analytics. Although the pursuit of self-knowledge and self-optimisation fundamentally depends on the organic body as the principal 'object of information', the means of sensemaking is increasingly outsourced to and performed by auxiliary codifying mechanisms that are adjudged to encompass greater degrees of validity and reliability. This raises important sociological questions pertaining to contemporary experiences of embodiment, especially the displacement of 'feeling representations' to digitised sensemaking infrastructures that become primary oracles of the objectivated body.

Methods

This study adopted an online ethnographic approach to analyse 'naturally occurring' qualitative material posted on the official QS website, in terms of presented narratives, statistics, and iconography. We were keen to investigate the language self-trackers use during their 'show and tell' confessions and the sentiments shared between presenter and audience, as well as visual representations of and responses to self-tracking practices/experiences. These accounts provided details pertinent to our interest in how and why people engage *with* and *through* digitised data, what data means to them, and how it was leveraged for personal development.

The sample comprised 30 videos, and featured the reflections of 5 female and 25 male self-trackers from predominantly professional and tech backgrounds in the U.S. Most of the excerpts were approximately seven to eight minutes in duration (Table 1). Each of these was fully transcribed and then coded in accordance with *inductive* (i.e. from the data) and *deductive* (i.e. from the literature) thematic categories. The approach adopted was similar to that of Choe, Lee, Lee, Pratt, and Kientz (2014) who purposively sampled 52 videos for analysis between January 2012 and April 2013. These authors used a two-part exclusion criterion requiring (1) that the speaker talked about their own data practices and (2) that the presentation contained a legible data visualisation for additional context. We copied this rubric, but applied it only to the most recent videos uploaded to the site when the research was conducted – that is, from August 2014 to July 2015. This allowed for an entirely new dataset to be analysed. The excerpts presented below were selected on the basis that they revealed important aspects of the interplay between self-tracked data, embodiment, and narratives of the self.

Online research can raise difficult ethical considerations, in terms of distinguishing what is public, from what is private, data, deciding whether informed consent need to be obtained from the research 'participants' given the lack of spatial and temporal proximity, and determining whether a researcher is obliged to disclose her identity. For the purpose of this preliminary research, the data utilised predominantly derive from the voluntary communicative acts of a 'networked public' (boyd, 2014, p. 5), and it is therefore treated in this spirit as a public asset and resource. Two semi-structured qualitative interviews were also conducted with individuals not affiliated with the QS, but who were enthusiastic users of self-tracking devices and personal analytic infrastructures. This was to produce a richer account of self/data relations, and to clarify issues not obtainable from the analysis of pre-recorded and thus circumscribed content.

The social life of self-tracking

The QS is an international collaboration of designers and users of self-tracking tools and mediums. Founded in 2007 by Gary Wolf and Kevin Kelly and comprising a worldwide network of approximately 43,000 self-trackers, QS organises regular conventions for self-trackers to transfer the knowledge they gleaned from their self-monitoring practices and experiences of digital data. They use a dedicated website to post information on

Table 1. QS video analysis matrix.

Self-tracker and self-tracking practice	Source
Anand Sharma: Aprilzero, Gyroscope, and Me	http://quantifiedself.com/2015/07/anand-sharma-april-zero-gyroscope/
Catha Mullen: Tracking My Financial Health	http://quantifiedself.com/2015/04/catha-mullen-tracking-financial-health/
Anna Nicanorova: My Year in Numbers	http://quantifiedself.com/2015/04/anna-nican-year-numbers/
Alice Pilgram: My Journey with Diabetes	http://quantifiedself.com/2015/04/alice-pilgram-journey-diabetes/
Gordon Bell: Every Beat of My Heart	http://quantifiedself.com/2015/03/gordon-bell-every-beat-heart/
Greg Kroleski: Six Years of Tracking My Time	http://quantifiedself.com/2015/02/greg-kroleski-six-years-tracking-time/
Paul La Fontaine: Heart Rate Variability and Flow	http://quantifiedself.com/2015/01/paul-lafontaine-heart-rate-variability-flow/
Sebastien Le Tuan: Tracking Punctuality	http://quantifiedself.com/2015/01/sebastien-le-tuan-tracking-punctuality/
Bill Schuller: The Quantified Talk	http://quantifiedself.com/2014/12/bill-schuller-quantified-talk/
Julie Price: 30lbs of Family Visits, Races, and Games	http://quantifiedself.com/2014/12/julie-price-30lbs-family-visits-races-games/
David Joerg: Building My Personal Operating System	http://quantifiedself.com/2014/12/david-joerg-building-personal-operating-system/
Greg Schwartz: Quantified Dating	http://quantifiedself.com/2014/12/greg-schwartz-quantified-dating/
Nan Shellabarger: 26 Years of Weight Tracking	http://quantifiedself.com/2014/11/nan-shellabarger-longterm-weight-tracking/
Ben Finn: Improving My Sleep	http://quantifiedself.com/2014/11/ben-finn-improving-sleep/
Cathal Gurrin: Me and My Log	http://quantifiedself.com/2014/11/cathal-gurrin-log/
Benjamin Bolland: What I Learned from Emotion Tracking	http://quantifiedself.com/2014/11/benjamin-bolland-learned-emotion-tracking/
Akshay Patil: Better Relationships Through Technology	http://quantifiedself.com/2014/11/akshay-patil-better-relationships-technology/
Jamie Williams: Exploring my Data	http://quantifiedself.com/2014/10/jamie-williams-exploring-data/
Tim Ngwena: My Music Listening Habits	http://quantifiedself.com/2014/10/tim-ngwena-music-listening-habits/
Shawn Dimantha: My Face, My Health	http://quantifiedself.com/2014/10/shawn-dimantha-face-health/
Ralph Pethica: Improving My Fitness With Genetics	http://quantifiedself.com/2014/10/ralph-pethica-improving-fitness-genetics/
Cliff Atkinson: Storyboarding the Psyche	http://quantifiedself.com/2014/10/cliff-atkinson-storyboarding-psyche/
Paul LaFontaine: Upset Every Other Minute	http://quantifiedself.com/2014/09/paul-lafontaine-every-minute/
Kouris Kalligas: Analyzing My Weight and Sleep	http://quantifiedself.com/2014/09/kouris-kalligas-analyzing-weight-sleep/
Lee Rogers: Why Annual Reporting	http://quantifiedself.com/2014/08/lee-rogers-annual-reporting/
Mark Drangsholt: Deciphering My Brain Fog	http://quantifiedself.com/2014/08/mark-drangsholt-deciphering-brain-fog/
Kevin Krejci: An Update on Tracking Parkinson's Disease	http://quantifiedself.com/2014/08/kevin-krejci-update-tracking-parkinsons/
Eric Boyd: Tracking My Daily Rhythm With a Nike FuelBand	http://quantifiedself.com/2014/08/eric-boyd-tracking-daily-rhythm-nike-fuelband/
Cors Brinkman: Lifelog as Self-Portrait	http://quantifiedself.com/2014/08/cors-brinkman-lifelog-self-portrait/
Philip Thomas on Building a Personal Dashboard	http://quantifiedself.com/2014/08/philip-thomas-building-personal-dashboard/

self-tracking techniques, practices, and events, and to embed the monitory activities of individual self-trackers within a broader community framework. As Kelly (2012) succinctly puts it, QS is principally about the pursuit of 'self-knowledge through numbers'. It is about individuals learning to read and inhabit their bodies in new ways through the mediums of data *and* audience feedback, but also to use such insight to reform entrenched habits and to enrich their life circumstances.

In contrast to concerns within scholarly circles about the surveillant capacities of sensor devices (Andrejevic & Gates, 2014), Kelly and Wolf highlight the participatory and empowering dimensions of self-tracking and data sharing practices. Prioritising the virtues of the entrepreneurial and reflexive self, self-trackers believe that data sharing repertoires provide a means to indirectly access opaque somatic processes and the unconscious self, and thereby to produce a blueprint of physiology and subjectivity that can be worked on and optimised. They hold and reify the belief that there is an affective layer of experience that can be detected and accessed through the medium of data. From this perspective, data function as a window and conduit to interiority, and provide the self-tracker with a data-driven mirror through which they can procure knowledge on what were previously indiscernible or unintelligible bodily processes. Such insight can then be used to manage their bodies – and perform embodied practices – in more efficient and effective ways.

Nafus and Sherman (2014, p. 1787) found QS meetups to be 'relatively coherent across sites', most encompassing a similar format and script. The theatrical 'show and tell' presentations are a customary feature of QS meetups, and these confessional monologues initiate a solidarity among self-trackers, in terms of presenters explaining to a susceptive audience how and why technologies were designed and selected, what the self-tracking program sought to reveal and what it actually exposed, and how it acted as a catalyst for further self-analysis and behavioural modification. As Sharon and Zandbergen (2016, p. 10) note,

> Standing on stage, self-trackers speak about painful episodes in their lives (depression, divorce, disease); they expose their dreams, their diary entries and their meditation practices, and they reveal minutiae about their physical ailments and their struggles with weight and mental well-being. Far from an aggregation of data-obsessed narcissists, then, what one witnesses here is closer to a confessional community, where numbers are used to 'confess' intimate details of personal lives to others.

It would be easy to surmise that the hyper-individualised self-tracker identity eclipses that of being a fellow 'Q-Selfer' member/participant. But we would argue in contrast that, for the reasons alluded to by Sharon and Zandbergen above, the QS audience – along with the 'dispersed audience' embedded in the implanted data-transmitting mechanisms – provides motivation not necessarily for initiating, but certainly for persevering with, self-tracking practices. For some, the impetus to self-track is socially driven and exceeds the exclusive quest for self-knowledge, reflecting desires instead to narrate personal experiences and stories in a public forum via the 'companion' medium of their data. The audience functions to validate the personal struggles and technical gadgetry of self-trackers, it supports potentially discrediting presentations of self, and affirms that the obsessive tracking of bodily experiences is normal and desirable. It helps institute a collective consciousness valorising practices of self-exposure, and it situates data-subjects in a dual role as *subjects* and *agents* of surveillance.

Of course, we realise there is a spectrum of affiliations to the organisation but we do not wish to enter into debates here as to whether or not the QS represents a comparable community for all its contributors. Instead, our concern is to accentuate the *social life* of data, the fact that digital devices and media infrastructures function to convert aspects of personal experience into a textual format that facilitates modes of dialogical exchange. In Kelly's (2009) view, data sharing is 'the mildest form of socialism', actuating experiences of comradeship and companionship, and serving 'as the foundation for higher levels of communal engagement'. For Lupton (2013b, p. 29), these behaviours are 'central to the web 2.0 age, in which sharing of data and other forms of content is valorised'. As she asserts, when individual trackers engage online or meet up in person, 'the quantified self becomes the quantified community' (Lupton, 2013b, p. 28).

The addictiveness of data

In an era of liquid modernity, the body is progressively characterised as being 'porous' and 'without limits' (Bauman, 2005, p. 93). This absence of frontier is epitomised, Bauman (2000, pp. 77–8) contends, by the cultural ideal of 'fitness' – which refers less to the actual physical condition of the body than to a biopolitical framing of it as deficient and in need of improvement. The notion of fitness is open-ended and delusive, and is personified by the maxim, 'however fit your body is – you could always make it fitter' (Bauman, 2005, p. 93). This way of conceptualising the body positions it as an ongoing project that demands the investment of attentiveness and labour, and the consumption of enrichment goods and services. Self-tracking practices are intrinsically bound to such logics. They are the outcome of technological development, discourses of self-reflexiveness, and efforts to optimise one's own life by exposing the body so that its component parts can be rendered legible and fixable (Lupton, 2013a, 2014a). The visualisation of interiority through the medium of digital data is key to such transformations in self-determination.

Ruckenstein (2014, p. 73) found participants in her research construing self-tracking as a 'catalyst for change'. Using data to orientate one's behaviour in this way evokes Foucault's (1988) seminal conceptualisation of *technologies of the self*. Technologies of the self are the mechanisms, ideas, and practices, from self-help manuals to medicines, that constitute the ways people engage in caring for the self. Engineering a stable sense of self entails looking *at* the body so as to 'objectivate' it, but also looking *beyond* the body for specialised techniques that, when leveraged, will help modulate it in desirable and productive ways. Such techniques typically conform to expert (of the political, medical, and commercial sort) discourses pertaining to the subjective management of well-being. More often than not, they operate in highly normative ways as modes of power that bring the errant or flawed self into line with governmental expectations and social conventions. Mutually related discourses of self-imperfection and self-improvement are common in the QS community, and they are specifically prevalent in the narratives expressed by those seeking to enhance their health states through the objectivating character of data. Data are fetishised to the point where they come – literally and metaphorically – to speak on behalf of the embodied referents they represent, and to provide the divine instruction, discipline, and impetus needed to enact a lifestyle intervention. They are in this sense a *medium of subjectivation*. Prosuming data reflects the internalisation of cultural obsessions with 'finding the self', with a view to managing it better via data-driven modes of knowing.

Data are construed as conduits for making meaningful alterations to daily routines and habits that are deemed harmful or irrational, and for maximising lived experiences of the body: to develop its capacities to think, feel, communicate, seduce, and act. In this way, practices of self-tracking and data accretion intersect with desires to enhance personal circumstances and to exert control over social trajectory. For example, Kevin, in his mid-50s and suffering from Parkinson's disease, exhibits a subjectivated narrative of data, where objectivated data patterns play a critical role in how he manages his chronic illness. He speaks of his wish to improve his overall quality of life through mutual practices of self-tracking and bodily datafication so that his enervative body is both conserved and operated in the most efficient ways possible:

> [The] main thing is to optimise productivity and quality of life … maximise productivity, type faster, work faster, run around the office faster, reduce stress … optimise routines … improve sleep results.

Likewise, Anand, who is in his mid-20s and has developed his own 'gyroscope' app to aggregate the various data traces from his everyday actions into a virtual 'event matrix' that records/visualises every moment of his life, told a QS audience:

> I wanted to fix my vitamin D levels, run faster, lower my heart rate, I wanted to be more productive … basically just become superman.

Anand highlights the importance of data in his pursuit of self-development, stating that 'actually tracking the stuff is really, really important, and the numbers are what kind of tell you what to do'. This technophilic account is intriguing for it reveals how data are subject to fetishisation, attributed with a veracity and transformative agency that comes, in a dialectical fashion, to wield a significant influence on how data-providers understand themselves and behave. Anand goes on to note,

> one thing I realised was that I got sick a few times, and I looked back on my logs, and my heart rates were way higher, like in the hundreds … So that was an interesting benchmark of figuring out, hey I'm sick, just from the numbers.

His data do not entirely override sensations deriving from his sensory faculties, but instead add a horizon of instruction to organise his quests for the acquisition of the appropriate biocapital that will boost his physiological performances, and thus supply him with a sense of achievement and validation.

Discourses of personal responsibility were also prevalent motives and outcomes in many of the other QS presentations. Kouris, in his late-30s and tracking his weight and sleep trends, pointed out that, 'it's important to find out what the data tells you, because then it's your choice to actually do something about it'. This kind of verbalisation attests how subjective attentiveness is outsourced to the data outputs to the point where forms of embodied knowledge are marginalised as unhelpful or untrustworthy, especially bodily signals, sensations, and intuitiveness. In the search for data-driven answers and directions, embodied consciousness is temporarily transferred from the interiorities and sensations of the body, to instead focus on their exteriorised representation as mediated visualisations.

In the context of QS, practices of self-tracking have a disciplinary and subjectivating quality. A key aspect of meetup events is the confessional admission where presenters disclose to a networked public the personal problem they sought to objectivate and address through data-driven analytics, the moment of epiphany when a detrimental habit or factor became apparent, and the responses they consequently mobilised. This ritual operates to reify the perceived need to engage in voluntary modes of self-surveillance while enrolling participants into conformist behaviours that pertain to dominant discourses of self-imperfection, metricisation, and improvement through the guise of data-driven visibility and self-directed autonomy. In Anand's case – where he deliberately made his personal data available for public scrutiny – a key inspiration was to receive 'motivational [read disciplinary] feedback' from a virtual audience: 'I built this just for myself … but I decided to put it up on the internet. There was no privacy, nothing is secret, everything I do is out there.' He proceeds to describe how exposing his self-tracked data impacted on his consequent behaviour:

> It changed my behaviour a lot. One thing I realised was I started showing off and running way longer … people also started emailing me telling me I'm a wuss and I should run more, which was really motivating. The idea of sharing everything turned out to be a really positive experience for me.

The networked audience became a source of stimulus for Anand, not only through its projected gaze, but also through its mediated interaction with him, inciting his desire to push himself harder and further on each run and thus materialise his aspiration of enhanced fitness and vitality. Similarly, when describing her tracking of type-II diabetes, Alice told the Bay Area meetup group how she aspired to make her health data-points available to both her primary care provider and family, as she felt the anticipated solidarities provided by this support team would keep her more focused on the 'burdensome' task of managing her illness. Alice's case attests how the existence of data proxies enable the exercise of discipline to be outsourced from the territories of the self to an external audience, albeit in her case a familial one:

> I'd like to be able to share this with my family, especially as I get older. They might want to know what's going on in my life especially when they're not nearby … And making sure they're helping me to keep honest and keep on top of what's going on.

As Bauman (2005, p. 17) contends, the elusive search for a stable identity in a liquid world means we have little choice but to look 'inside of ourselves'. Both in the context of the QS community in general and the interviewees in particular, self-trackers expressed a strong desire to increase the supply of data relating to their bodies. The will for greater self-knowledge and bodily enlightenment was framed around an inherent dissatisfaction with – and distrust of – the sensing, feeling, and intuitive organic body as a bounded instrument of illumination and as a vehicle of change. It was grounded instead in the belief that an increase in the quantity and quality of data *about* that body could improve embodied wellness. This doctrinal perception encourages the self-tracker to transcend the perceived limitations of biological forms of sensing. The paradoxical process of *looking beyond* – while simultaneously *looking at* – the body creates the preference for implementing ambient recording devices that can objectivate corporeality in its natural and non-contrived state, and in an unfiltered way that does not invalidate the objectivity of the results. Such multi-layered and multi-mediated looking is founded on ontological and epistemological assumptions. It implicitly construes devices as untainted bearers of truth and bodies as pure 'objects of information', as providing stable (i.e. datafiable) reference points for the sourcing of the required knowledge. There is a tacit appreciation that the nature of interiorised affects cannot be derived from direct consciousness alone and the resultant difficulties of approaching the object of investigation (the body/self) as a subjectivated inhabitant. They must instead be exteriorised through the medium of digital data.

Kate, a university student who engaged in sleep-tracking to help manage a chronic condition, described how she wanted to measure variables other than sleep for greater contextual awareness of illness trigger factors, a task she felt her conscious mind alone could not achieve: 'I would definitely prefer to be tracking mood during the day; that would actually be useful ... it would just be one more layer to have. And you can never have enough data.' As Whitson (2013, p. 175) notes, 'quantification of the self allows us to replace the holes in our memories and the vagaries of our intuition' with the apparent objectivity and perspicacity of data-based knowledge, a techno-driven movement that makes instinctual powers of the body–mind progressively more peripheral and obsolescent as sources of enlightenment, awareness, edification, and truth. In this deterministic turn to processes of externalisation and objectivation, knowledge of the body/self is only validated if it appears *outside* of the body/self, especially in the form of a multiplex data visualisation.

Bauman (2005, p. 80) argues that liquid modernity is defined by the elusive pursuit of fulfilment, with seduction located more within the 'promise of satisfaction' than the 'experience of satisfaction' itself. This is typified in the logic of consumer societies where immediate contentment is subordinated by promises of eternal happiness (Bauman, 2005, p. 83). Device-sensed data are seen to satisfy our desires to 'know' more about ourselves than what the body (and its biological sensors) alone can tender, yet they also function to instil a normative and normalising perception that additional flows of data will reveal further truths about selfhood, and its ecological interdependencies. This perception subscribes to a techno-utopic impression that self-understanding cannot be established via embodied introspection and meditation alone, requiring instead technological platforms that can excavate and present the surfaces and depths of the self without subjectifying biases corrupting processes of interpretation. This renders the satisfaction of each datafied insight marginal to the potential of future data-driven self-knowledge, thus perpetuating an addictive striving for the creation of additional data from within. A number of QS speakers framed this impulse as an 'obsession', alluding to the ephemeral satisfaction derived from visualised data that is prosumed and then quickly discarded as dated or obsolete, or considered only intelligible when amalgamated with supplementary data-points.

Becoming with data

Self-tracked data are used as a medium to generate stories *for* and *about* the body/self. But equally, the digital devices and data flows themselves provide their own unique forms of authorship. In this way, the data-subject translates the data just as the data apps and outputs translate the actions of the self-tracker. In other words, data-subjects and their data proxies are mutually engaged in relational interplays and entanglements, they *become with* one another and mediate how each appears in specific actor-networks (Smith, 2016). They both contribute in variable measure to a multi-agent and multi-mediated body/self/data dialogue. As Klauser and Albrechtslund (2014, p. 278) note, datafying the self

> is related to describing, signifying or interpreting the self in terms of material facts ... stories and metaphors ... From this perspective, quantification is about modes of presenting and structuring an account of the self, for example as a narrative configuration.

Research by Lomborg and Frandsen (2015) has shown how self-tracking as a social and cultural practice is fundamentally communicative in format and nature. Applying this framework to those participating in self-tracking can help us better understand how data is used in manifold ways to (a) inform on the body/self, (b) motivate and stimulate behaviours, and (c) construct social narratives of health. The self-tracker produces and defines the data as much as the data objectivates and subjectivates the body/self.

Commonly referred to as 'nudges', that is, vibrations when a certain number of steps are taken or audio alerts reminding device-bearers to exercise, the ability of devices to autonomously communicate to the user in real time and structure their consequent actions is becoming a common feature of self-tracking experiences (Lupton, 2015b, p. 1351). These nudges play a pivotal role in orchestrating – that is, incentivising, pressurising, and automating – health-related behaviours in a 'techno-body' symbiosis. Alice, for example, spoke proudly about how her digital tracking system dispatches automated text messages to remind her to measure her blood sugar level:

> I had to track the highs and the lows. I had to be conscientious about the changes happening in my body … I can see a nice graph telling me I've been doing a good job or not doing a good job.

Alice's self-tracking is emblematic of Lupton's (2013a) 'digitally engaged patient', where citizens are expected to use portable consumer technologies to serve biopolitical ends: to develop bodily expertise for leveraging on themselves to improve levels of desirability, vitality, and productivity. Her narrative also reveals the degree to which bodily attentiveness is devolved from embodied sentience to an a digitising that is not subject to bouts of amnesia, stress, or intoxication. As a result, these technologies help cultivate a self-reflexive subject who is aware of the deficiencies of her/his consciousness and sensorium, and the corollary need to maintain the body via a repertoire of mandated behaviours that are prompted by the automated monitoring regimes of machinic bioproxies. Alice is not only adhering to dominant discourses which shift the burden of healthcare onto the individual, but is also reinforcing popular notions of data as being unfiltered sources of truth, while consequently reifying perceptions of embodied sentience as untrustworthy. Yet for Alice, this shift was empowering, she felt reassured from being able to reclaim control over the management of a condition that had previously felt intractable.

In other cases, this affective dialogue between machine and person is not as straightforward. Presenting to the Bay Area QS meetup group, Paul, a male in his mid-50s, described his efforts to track what he calls his 'upsets' – which translate as intense sensations of stress. Rather than seek to directly address the complex social causes of his embodied distress, Paul's narration reveals the way that self-trackers sometimes opt to manage the expression of symptoms through an amalgam of technical means and techno-ideals. Using a wearable heart rate monitor to map when he entered into these intensities, the device would signal to him by emitting a flashing red light and an accompanying alert. As Paul describes:

> When the machine told me I was upset, I would then talk into my audio recorder … so I could actually hear the way I got myself out of it [through breathing and calming utterances].

Paul initially doubted the reliability of the device's feedback loop, 'When I first started using it, when it would flash red I would sit there and debate the machine – "you can't be right?!" – I started calling it "freakback"'. Yet by the end of his self-tracking experience, Paul came 'to accept the readings' as objective indicators of his affective state. In this sense, Paul put the technology's reading of himself above his own intuitive cognition. In this way, human–machine relationalities can produce dialectics that rotate on variant definitions of feeling, where human-based intuition is confronted with machine-based learning. This entanglement of meanings, those generated by the mutual actions of subjects and objects, is a common one in discussions of digital data. A key concern is that with the increasing transfer of power to machine-based algorithms and the situation of such infra-structures within state and corporate fields, the embodied actors providing the data get excluded and estranged from the codifications that come to either structure their everyday repertoires or 'nudge' them to specific ends (Klauser & Albrechtslund, 2014, p. 278).

While data are often presented as irrefutable, in many instances, self-quantification operates in tandem with sensory experiences to produce emergent forms of social practice. As a result, data proxies can tender not only a digital artefact for objectivation, but also represent a medium to be negotiated with in processes of subjectivation (Lupton, 2012, p. 237). At times, their existence and content create a disconnect between how someone *should* feel, and how they *actually* feel. In particular, certain self-trackers described how data-based measures failed to fully reflect the richness of phenomenological experience. Sara, a university student, described how her unbodied sleep-tracking app did not ade-quately reflect her embodied experiences of sleep and fatigue:

> It tells you about that sleep for the night, and I don't think it always reflects how you feel … because you could have had a relaxed day, but the app would still say you've had a restless sleep.

Importantly, this ongoing negotiation between self-trackers and their unbodied data exhaust occurs even in cases where the data is interpreted as an accurate reflection of lived experience. For example, Kate's description of her sleep data reveals a deeply ambig-uous relation, where the virtualised data-archive had the capacity to produce simultaneous goods and bads depending on what it conveyed and the resultant meaning she attributed to it:

> You know, if it says 78% sleep quality last night, that is pretty good for me … It's kind of self-manipulative, I'll be like, 'oh I must have slept well, I'm going to have a good day today'.

And yet, for Kate, a restless sleep pattern was correlated with a higher risk of experiencing a seizure, a data-mediated reality that caused her considerable embodied distress. Moreover, there were other visualisations where despite the data indicating a stable sleep pattern, she subsequently suffered a seizure, and a breakdown in data-based trust ensued. As she describes: 'those are the kind of … days where I'm more likely to not then use the app again'. In addition, she disclosed that she avoids looking at the data on the days following a seizure: 'I don't want to see it.' When asked to explain this choice, she described a feeling of data overload: 'just knowing pretty much … I don't want to deal with this'. As Kate negotiates with her data exhaust on a daily basis, she walks a fine line between what the proxy actually communicates, what she wants to see/hear, and what she then experiences on the bodily register.

Self-tracking with digital data, particularly in the case of QS, is a social and relational practice, as engaging with personal data becomes akin to a performative event (Lomborg &

Frandsen, 2015; Lupton, 2014a). As Lupton (2014a, p. 9) contends, self-tracking is about not only the 'stories people tell themselves' through their data, but also the stories and types of selves they exhibit publically. In various presentations, QS speakers describe how they started self-tracking for health reasons and then started using the data to develop a more informed and coherent biography. For example, Lee, a serial lifelogger in his mid-30s, aggregated data-points into an annual report visualisation which helped him to escape the myopia of embodied memory and to better narrate his year as a totality:

> When you're creating a book for somebody else to look at, you analyse the data in a different way to how you would have done before ... I also started a narrative of my findings. This storytelling allowed me to translate the data into a better representation of the kind of person I was that year.

Similarly Cors, a visual arts student, converted a year's worth of self-portraits into an amalgamated data visualisation as a way to track, but also present, his annual mental health report. For Cors, his exteriorised data allowed him to 'convey a personal story' – an interiority – which captured how his sensory experience of well-being was in fact ecologically related, being, and contingent on the status of his personal relationships and on environmental fluctuations. By creating a visually engaging graphic through which self-trackers like Cors communicate their experiences, 'self-knowledge and self-expression' is simultaneously achieved (Lupton, 2014a, p. 12). In these examples, self-tracking becomes not only a practice of self-monitoring and data-driven introspection, but also a mode of 'communicating dimensions of the self using visual or other material based on one's data' (Lupton 2013b, p. 29). Therefore, the collective aspect of the QS is integral to bringing discrete people together through a shared medium, a factor which initiates a dialogue between the self, its data Other, and a networked audience.

Conclusion

The field of personal and public healthcare has become a terrain where networked digital sensors and techno-bodied subjects are engaged in mutual dialogues: relationalities that are fundamentally re-shaping conventional conceptualisations of embodiment, health, and illness. We have pointed to some of the complex interplays that are occurring in this field, interplays that incorporate the reciprocal interactivity between digitised devices and media infrastructures, modes of expertise, embodied subjects, data flows and visualisations. What seems evident is that the unbodied biotexts visualised via self-tracking practices are increasingly mediating how data-providers understand, experience, and inhabit the objectivated territories of their bodies. This opens up a new politics of the body which, as we have seen, can have empowering and disempowering dimensions, as data transmissions come to act as both enabling and constraining forces in the production of bodily and social relations. We have pointed to the way in which intuition is being outsourced to, if not displaced by, the medium of unbodied data. It is this objectivated facility that is increasingly used as an intuitive device for orientating behavioural decisions as they relate to bodily maintenance. Key to understanding the implications of this emergent social practice is the initiation of more participatory empirical studies which give prominence to the social meanings that data both convey and embody as referents and mediums of the subject.

Acknowledgements

We wish to thank the two reviewers and Deborah Lupton for their excellent and instructive comments on an earlier draft of this paper. We also wish to thank Norma Smith for her diligence in proofreading this paper.

Disclosure statement

No potential conflict of interest was reported by the authors.

References

Andrejevic, M., & Gates, K. (2014). Editorial big data surveillance: Introduction. *Surveillance & Society, 12*(2), 185–196.
Bauman, Z. (2000). *Liquid modernity.* Cambridge: Polity Press.
Bauman, Z. (2005). *Liquid life.* Cambridge: Polity Press.
Beck, U., Giddens, A., & Lash, S. (1994). *Reflexive modernization: Politics, tradition and aesthetics in the modern social order.* Cambridge: Polity Press.
Berger, P., & Luckmann, T. (1966). *The social construction of reality: A treatise in the sociology of knowledge.* London: Penguin.
boyd, d. (2014). *It's complicated: The social lives of networked teens.* New Haven, CT: Yale University Press.
Choe, E. K., Lee, N. B., Lee, B., Pratt, W., & Kientz, J. A. (2014). Understanding quantified-selfers' practices in collecting and exploring personal data. In *Proceedings of the 32nd Annual ACM Conference on Human Factors in Computing Systems* (pp. 1143–1152). Toronto: ACM Press. http://dx.doi.org/10.1145/2556288.2557372
Dalton, C., & Thatcher, J. (2014). What does a critical data studies look like, and why do we care? Seven points for a critical approach to 'big data'. *Society and Space.* Retrieved June 6, 2015, from http://societyandspace.com/material/commentaries/craig-dalton-and-jim-thatcher-what-does-a-critical-data-studies-look-like-and-why-do-we-care-seven-points-for-a-critical-approach-to-big-data
Foucault, M. (1988). Technologies of the self. In L. H. Martin, H. Gutman, & P. H. Hutton (Eds.), *Technologies of the self: A seminar with Michel Foucault* (pp. 16–49). Amherst: University of Massachusetts Press.
French, M., & Smith, G. J. D. (2013). Health surveillance: New modes of monitoring bodies, populations, and polities. *Critical Public Health, 23*(4), 383–392. doi:10.1080/09581596.2013.838210
Hortensius, J., Kars, M. C., Wierenga, W. S., Kleefstra, N., Bilo, H. J., & van der Bijl, J. J. (2012). Perspectives of patients with type 1 or insulin-treated type 2 diabetes on self-monitoring of blood glucose: A qualitative study. *BMC Public Health, 12*(1), 1–11.
Kelly, K. (2009). The new socialism. Retrieved November 15, 2015, from http://www.wired.co.uk/magazine/archive/2009/07/features/the-new-socialism
Kelly, K. (2012). Kevin Kelly on the history and future of QS. Retrieved November 16, 2015, from http://quantifiedself.com/2012/10/kevin-kelly-on-the-history-and-future-of-qs
Klauser, F. R., & Albrechtslund, A. (2014). From self-tracking to smart urban infrastructures: Towards an interdisciplinary research agenda on big data. *Surveillance and Society, 12*(2), 273–286.

Lomborg, S., & Frandsen, K. (2015). Self-tracking as communication. *Information, Communication & Society, 18*, 1–13. doi:10.1177/1368431006065717

Lupton, D. (2012). M-health and health promotion: The digital cyborg and surveillance society. *Social Theory & Health, 10*(3), 229–244.

Lupton, D. (2013a). The digitally engaged patient: Self-monitoring and self-care in the digital health era. *Social Theory & Health, 11*(3), 256–270. doi:10.1057/sth.2013.10

Lupton, D. (2013b). Understanding the human machine. *IEEE Technology and Society Magazine, 32*(4), 25–30. doi:10.1109/MTS.2013.2286431

Lupton, D. (2014a). You are your data: Self-tracking practices and concepts of data. Retrieved November 10, 2015, from http://papers.ssrn.com/sol3/papers.cfm?abstract_id=2534211

Lupton, D. (2014b). *Self-tracking modes: Reflexive self-monitoring and data practices.* Paper given at the 'Imminent Citizenships: Personhood and Identity Politics in the Informatic Age' workshop, ANU, Canberra. Retrieved November 15, 2015, from http://papers.ssrn.com/sol3/papers.cfm?abstract_id=2483549

Lupton, D. (2015a). Quantified sex: A critical analysis of sexual and reproductive self-tracking using apps. *Culture, Health & Sexuality, 17*(4), 440–453. doi:10.1080/13691058.2014.920528

Lupton, D. (2015b). Critical perspectives on digital health technologies. *Sociology Compass, 8*(12), 1344–1359. doi:0.1111/soc4.12226

Nafus, D., & Sherman, J. (2014). This one does not go up to 11: The quantified self movement as an alternative big data practice. *International Journal of Communication, 8*(1), 1784–1794.

Ruckenstein, M. (2014). Visualized and interacted life: Personal analytics and engagements with data doubles. *Societies, 4*(1), 68–84. doi:10.3390/soc4010068

Sharon, T., & Zandbergen, D. (2016). From data fetishism to quantifying selves: Self-tracking practices and the other values of data. *New Media & Society.* doi:10.1177/1461444816636090

Smarr, L. (2012). Quantifying your body: A how-to guide from a systems biology perspective. *Biotechnology Journal, 7*(8), 980–991. doi:10.1002/biot.201100495

Smith, G. J. D. (2016). Surveillance, data and embodiment: On the work of being watched. *Body & Society, 22*(2), 108–139. doi:10.1177/1357034X15623622

Swan, M. (2009). Emerging patient-driven health care models: An examination of health social networks, consumer personalized medicine and quantified self-tracking. *International Journal of Environmental Research and Public Health, 6*(2), 492–525.

Whitson, J. R. (2013). Gaming the quantified self. *Surveillance & Society, 11*(1/2), 163–176.

Wolf, G. (2010). The data-driven life. Retrieved March 13, 2016, from http://www.nytimes.com/2010/05/02/magazine/02self-measurement-t.html

Social rhythms of the heart

Mika Pantzar, Minna Ruckenstein and Veera Mustonen

ABSTRACT

A long-term research focus on the temporality of everyday life has become revitalised with new tracking technologies that allow methodological experimentation and innovation. This article approaches rhythms of daily lives with heart-rate variability measurements that use algorithms to discover physiological stress and recovery. In the spirit of the 'social life of methods' approach, we aggregated individual data ($n = 35$) in order to uncover temporal rhythms of daily lives. The visualisation of the aggregated data suggests both daily and weekly patterns. Daily stress was at its highest in the mornings and around eight o'clock in the evening. Weekend stress patterns were dissimilar, indicating a stress peak in the early afternoon especially for men. In addition to discussing our explorations using quantitative data, the more general aim of the article is to explore the potential of new digital and mobile physiological tracking technologies for contextualising the individual in the everyday.

In a place of collection of fixed things, you will follow each *being*, each *body*, as having its own time above the whole. Each one therefore having its place, its rhythm, with its recent past, a foreseeable and a distant future. (Lefebvre, 2004, p. 31)

The hypothesis of this article is that the human heart beats not only as part of the nervous system, but also as part of social life. We depart from the notion that the regular rhythms of everyday life, such as collective eating and resting times, result from millions of seemingly separate time fragments, moments and episodes. According to Lefebvre (2004), a rhythm analyst sees rhythms everywhere in society. Listening to the sounds of the human body, cities and buildings as if he were listening to a symphony orchestra, and putting all his senses to work on diverse data and different fields of science, the analyst learns to recognise the diversity, repetition and forms of everyday life (Lefebvre, 2004, pp. 21–31).

Time, and its measuring and scheduling, are continually being socially re-ordered and adapted, a phenomenon which Thompson (1967) suggests is primarily linked to the deepening division of labour in society. Recent practice-oriented research (e.g. Pantzar &

Shove, 2010; Schatzki, 2010), on the other hand, has examined temporal regularities in terms of network-like interaction relations and feedbacks. Thus in addition to a focus on empirical time use, time-use research has increasingly become interested in the rhythms of everyday life (Gershuny, 2000; Pantzar, 2010; Ruckenstein, 2013; Southerton, 2003, 2006). As far as we know, physiological stress research and sociologically oriented rhythm analysis have not yet joined forces, although the research project discussed here specifically strives towards this end. The first endeavour is to describe the rhythms of everyday life through a novel means of visualisation, termed here the 'digital electrocardio-gram', a goal that resonates with the manner in which the details and dynamics of a gal-loping horse or a running human were first successfully captured on film and identified 150 years ago (see Bender & Marinar, 2010). We present an experimental research design wherein we tried to identify and visually capture social rhythms, especially those of stress and recovery, by measuring variations in electrical heart signals among 36 Finnish people.

The second research objective was to explore the potential of physiological tracking technologies in viewing the human as a biosocial entity. We found inspiration for research into the social rhythms of the heart in Rose's (2013, pp. 19–20) assertion:

> [I]t is clear that links will not be in terms of the relations of 'body' and 'society' – those enti-cing yet illusory totalities – but at a different scale. Not in terms of 'the body' or 'the brain' as coherent systems enclosed by a boundary of skin, but of bodies and brains as multiplicities, of the coexistence and symbiosis of multiple entities from bacterial flora in the gut, to the proliferation of neurons in the brain, each in multiple connections with milieux, internal and external, inorganic, organic, vital, historical, cultural, human. Distributed capacities in milieux which vital organisms themselves partly create and which in turn create them and their capacities.

This emphasis on the coexistencies of the external and internal, with attention paid to the forces of vitality, resonates with the new materialist theory focusing on 'choreographies of becoming' (Coole & Frost, 2010, p. 10), which proposes that no definitive division or break exists between living and material systems. Significantly, digital tracking devices have made it possible to apply doctrines of vitality and becoming in empirical research. Self-tracking can link together phenomena that have previously been regarded as isolated, such as the use of time and physiological reactions. This may also enable us to go past and beyond the juxtaposition between the biological and the social because, importantly, as our study demon-strates, the rhythms of individual hearts and society coexist and resonate with each other.

The fact that solutions for monitoring human physiology and activities have recently been vigorously developed in different parts of the world (e.g. Lupton, 2012, 2015; Swan, 2012, 2013), opens a lot of room for methodological experimentation. In practice this can be seen as an attempt to combine very different kinds of data in research exper-iments, taking a general curiosity-driven approach (DeLyser & Sui, 2012) which challenges the line between qualitative and quantitative research. Somewhat paradoxically, the expan-sion of measuring technologies in the social sciences to new spheres of life may also mean a narrowing of space for evidence-based truths and instrumental positivism, meanwhile providing added momentum to the performativity and expressivity of quantified data (Ruppert, Law, & Savage, 2013; Savage, 2013). In the section below, we briefly examine the historical and medical foundations of understandings of stress in humans before exploring the most thought-provoking results of our quantitative study.

Defining and measuring stress

The first writings on the stress to humans caused by a rapidly changing society began to appear in the early stages of industrialisation in the late eighteenth century (Rosa, 2003) when pre-modern industrialisation and its effects on people's endurance were becoming a source of concern among doctors. At that time, the term 'stress' still mainly referred to the concept of fracture point in the field of physics, however, and it was not until the twentieth century that the concept became part of biological, psychological and cybernetic terminology. An understanding that emphasised the balance of the nervous system (homeostasis) gained ground after World War II, as doctors started to conceive of the long-term stress suffered by soldiers on the battlefront as the effects of imbalance in the nervous system (Hinkle, 1974; Kugelman, 1992; Selye, 1973).

Today stress regulation is seen as being based on network-like mechanisms and further work has been conducted on this theory by an extensive group of researchers who have tried to find a sufficiently general definition for stress through animal testing (Koolhaas et al., 2011). According to their findings, stress comprises a state where the requirements of the environment exceed the capacity of the homeostatic regulatory system of any organism. Consequently, the major causes and manifestations of stress are connected to situations of uncontrollability and unpredictability, meaning that it is also important to understand the environment and changes in living conditions, as well as internal dynamics, in a dialogical relation to lived life and physiological processes (Koolhaas et al., 2011). This observation inspires the extension of attention, among humans as well as animals, from biological processes to social processes. One could, on the one hand, say that increased complexity and developments in the division of labour have led to a situation where an individual's chances to affect the terms of her/his own existence have become too small (anomia/alienation), thereby leading to stress. On the other hand, stress can be produced when an individual has too many things to control and too little security (values, norms) to be able to produce order (Hinkle, 1974).

In current stress research, the prevailing theories emphasise interaction between the individual and the environment. Without homeostatic mechanisms (hormones, etc.), the balance is shaken and potential health risks are realised as illnesses. As Lefebvre has pointed out, regularly repeated rhythms, at individual and collective levels, are an expression of interlinked routines and practices. In our research design, we follow Lefebvre, working on the principle that people have to adjust to other people's rhythms, a process which involves tension, something that may be reflected on the stress data. As discussed below, our results do support the view that stress is connected to conflicting pressures in the environment and the shocks and surprises that life engenders: in a word, 'arrhythmia'. Stress is an essential part of life, comprising an adjusting mechanism in the human body, and not harmful as such. It can, however, be risky if the heart does not recover from that state. In the following sections, we briefly explore our research design based on heart-rate variability (HRV) measurement.

Methodological considerations

Our research was centrally affected by the fact that we found ourselves taking part in a pre-prepared and well-resourced technology research program that emphasised a normative view of the health behaviour of individuals, mainly aiming to demonstrate that self-tracking technologies promote behaviour change; thus parts of the research design were instrumental and solution oriented. Yet, as explained below, we were able to expand the aims of the research by gathering, along with quantitative stress data, personal accounts of stress and recovery connected to certain moments and activities, in both real time and afterwards, by interviewing our test subjects and discussing their diaries and HRV measurement data with them.

The measuring device used in the study, developed by a Finnish company, Firstbeat Technologies (est. 2002), utilises a technical calculation algorithm to measure stress and recovery based on heart beat and HRV. The key motivation for taking advantage of this type of technology for measuring stress in a research design such as ours is its ease of application compared to assessments based, for example, on measuring the levels of stress hormones in saliva (Semmer, Grebner, & Elfering, 2004) or by monitoring blood pressure (Heaphy & Dutton, 2008). The representation of stress has crucially changed due to new memory-equipped sensory technologies that measure and record HRV. HRV calculation is based on variation of time in milliseconds between two heartbeats and importantly, makes no separation between 'good' and 'bad' stress. Instead, HRV reveals movements and changes between physiological recovery and stress. A change in HRV addresses and reflects the ability of the heart to adjust to changes in external conditions (Acharya, Joseph, Kannathal, Lim, & Suri, 2006; Uusitalo et al., 2011): to put it very simply, the underlying assumption of HRV analysis is that the more stressed the heart, the less it reacts to external conditions, something which is of particular interest when the cause of stress is no longer present (Kettunen, 1999) – that is, when HRV is low yet the pulse is higher than is considered normal. After an athlete has over-trained, for example, or after the high consumption of alcohol, periods are often produced characterised by this state of hormonal imbalance in the nervous system.

The quantitative research data consists of heart-rate measurements among a voluntary test group, comprising healthy, urban and physically active subjects, most of whom were employed, and aged between 28 and 52. The material was gathered in March and May 2012, with each of the two rounds comprising an average eight days of HRV measurement.[1] In the first period we recruited 20 participants, adding a further sample of 20 for the second period. Four of the subjects took part in both rounds and the test results of one of the participants were corrupted, so the experiment culminated in 35 individual participants who were recruited through a number of channels: posting invitations on social media sites, contacting sports teams and snowballing. People with a systematic and disciplined relationship to sports and exercise, or an interest in self-tracking technologies, are particularly drawn to this type of research, and one-third of our total research participants were active in their chosen sports at least four times a week. For the second round, we deliberately targeted subjects who were less engaged with exercise, inviting, for instance, artists, start-up entrepreneurs and mothers of small children to participate. The test subjects gave us their approval to analyse and present their individual data, but we have anonymised it nonetheless.

After the monitoring period, the subjects received an illustrated report based on Firstbeat HEALTH-software analysis of their HRV, including their own entries about everyday doings. The colours on the report represent stress and recovery measurements. We encouraged the participants to also write their own detailed diary entries during the monitoring period in order to provide a more contextual account of what the self-measuring data could reveal. The participants could freely decide whether they wanted to write in their diaries and what they wanted to share with us (see Ruckenstein, 2014). The Firstbeat report, additional diary entries and interviews after the monitoring period allowed the exploration of possible discrepancies between the HRV data and people's daily experiences of stress and recovery. Because of the many possible interpretations of stress and recovery represented in the report, we arranged sessions, with five to eight participants in each, in which the participants could discuss the stress peaks and recoveries depicted in the images (see Ruckenstein, 2014). These discussions brought to the fore that the information supplied both supported people's experiences of stress and recovery, but also departed from them. In order to understand better the possible discrepancies between reported measuring data and people's subjective experiences, we identified in people's self-reported diaries and interviews incidents (in our material a total of 169) that were characterised by an exceptionally high level of stress or recovery: with a predefined interest, these were the only kinds of incidents that we explored. We return in the end of the article to discuss findings based on those incidents, where stress or recovery was revealed in talk but not by the heart.

The physiological assumptions on which the Firstbeat summary is based rely on certain algorithms and therefore cannot be considered absolute in any way. We accepted Firstbeat Technology's algorithm, developed for measuring stress and recovery, as sufficiently valid for our research purposes, while remaining aware that scientific debate is still actively underway on the connection between HRV and stress. We did, however, diverge from Firstbeat's conventions of measuring stress: our follow-up period was longer than the company standard three days and we were not primarily interested in variations in states of stress at an individual level but, rather, in shared and collective times of stress and in recovery. Ultimately, our research project produced a matrix of tens of millions of observations, which would have been difficult to approach and analyse without the visual user interface, specially developed for the purpose, that enabled us to aggregate data and to compare different physiological states and individuals during different time periods. The crucial aspect of the developed visual tool was its capacity to depict alternative scenarios and events, and to produce numerous iterations for working with, and interpreting, the data.

By visually examining HRV within our test group, we deliberately emphasise the openness of our findings to interpretation (Andersson, Nafus, Rattenbury, & Aipperspach, 2009; Bender & Marinar, 2010; Edwards, Harvey, & Wade, 2010), while also following the conventions of representation in time-use research (Michelson, 2005), chronobiology (Foster & Kreitzman, 2004) and time geography (Ellegård & Vilhelmson, 2004), where visual analysis has traditionally played a central role. In the subsequent section, we examine some of the general features of physical and psychological stress in the weekly and daily rhythms of our test subjects. We also briefly reflect on reasons for the differences they exhibit by considering background variables that may affect stress levels. Following this, we reflect on the avenues that research results based on physiological measurement may open for social research.

Empirical findings

Daily and weekly stress rhythms

Daily stress calculated from the entire body of data, including both weekdays and weekends, was at its highest in the mornings and at around 8 pm in the evenings (Figure 1). On average, daily stress seemed to be at its lowest around 11 am and 5 pm. As we will later see, these times (which are possibly related to customary Finnish meal times) also stand out in the framework of recovery. A third stress peak in the day generally occurs in the afternoon, around 3 pm. It is noteworthy that daytime (on working days) appears, roughly viewed, to be less stressful among our test subjects than evenings. This conclusion is further confirmed when 15-minute intervals exceeding twice the average stress levels for this period of time are brought into focus. This calculative solution (emphasising highest stress levels) seems to work better when the starting point of the research is the common conception of stress as an especially strenuous period.

Thus, the average day of our test subjects seems to be divided by stress periods that occur in the morning, the afternoon and the evening. Could it be that transitions (e.g. to and from work) cause stress? Could stress in the evenings be connected to physical

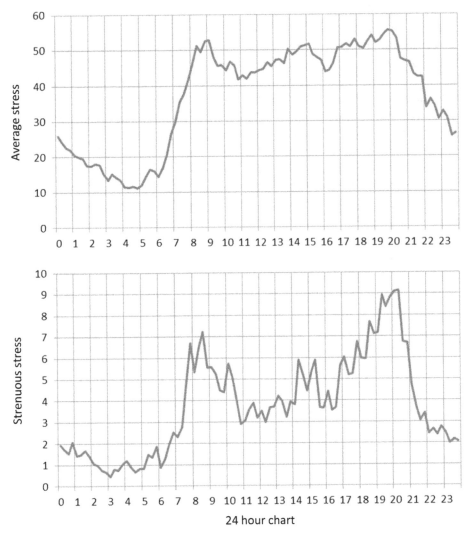

Figure 1. Daily stress. Upper: Average stress values for all the test subjects in 15-minute intervals (measured for each as the share of seconds that exceed the average in each 15-minute interval). Lower: percentage of seconds of stress more than twice as high as the average in 15-minute periods. The 15-minute interval of each test subject is compared to their personal average over approximately 10-day periods.

activity or the tensions of family life? In order to understand the underlying reasons for the results, we next remove the effect of weekdays from the figure, then briefly describe how the test subjects' background (gender, age) affects the stress profile.

As expected, the stress profiles for weekends and weekdays were different (Figure 2). In other words, stress peaks in the mornings and evenings are apparently connected to weekdays, while afternoon stress peaks seem to be connected to weekends. The significance tests also showed substantial variation in stress levels that correlated with the day of the week and the time of day. The overall picture becomes even clearer when we examine the weekly rhythm of stress among our test subjects by gender (Figures 3 and 4). Although the stress levels for both women and men were, overall, very low on Saturdays, there was a stress peak on Saturday afternoons, especially among the men.

To enable comparison, we divided the test subjects into groups of approximately the same size according the following criteria: age (24–33 and 34–52), body mass index (BMI) (19–23 and 24–32) and gender (female/$N = 20$, male/$N = 15$). In light of physiological research, it could be expected that, for example, age or poor physical condition might increase the average stress level (i.e. reduce HRV). Roughly assessed, however, the effects of age or BMI were rather small among our test group, though the impact of physical activity was more notable. Those of our test subjects who were more physically active experienced fewer extreme occasions of stress in the evenings, while extreme stress was divided equally throughout the day among the more sedentary people. We also assessed the effect of having children on the rhythm of stress by comparing those test subjects who had children ($n = 20$) to those who did not ($n = 15$), finding, on average, somewhat higher levels among those who had children, although variations in the stress level were higher among those without.

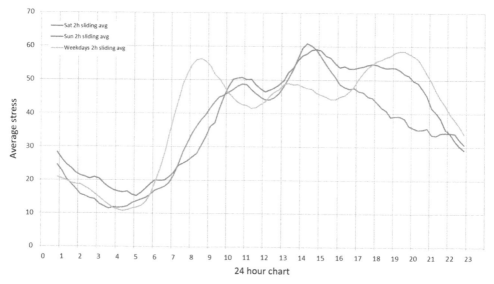

Figure 2. Stress during weekends vs. weekdays (share of seconds exceeding the stress average in 15-minute intervals.
Note: For example, from 8 am to 8.15 am, 53% of the observations per second were higher than the average.

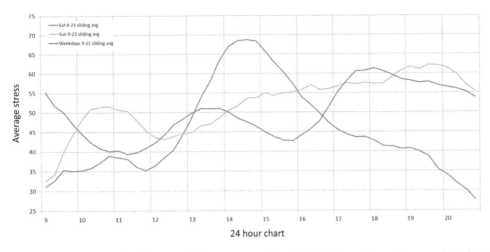

Figure 3. Stress on weekends vs. weekdays among male subjects (share of seconds exceeding the personal stress average in 15-minute intervals).

Daily and weekly rhythm of recovery

As could be expected, night time was the most significant period of recovery for our test subjects with only a little recovery taking place during the day, although the picture changes when we examine the recovery profile between 9 am and 9 pm (Figure 5). There is again a marked difference between weekends and weekdays. On weekdays, recovery seems to be concentrated around lunch and dinner times, and late evenings, while on Saturdays and Sundays, the late afternoon and especially evenings exhibit the most marked recovery periods. In common with the stress profile, recovery on weekends is at its lowest in the afternoon, around 3 pm. Overall, the day (and night) showing the highest recovery levels was Saturday.

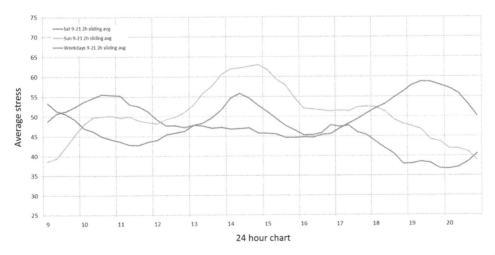

Figure 4. Stress on weekends vs. weekdays among female subjects (share of seconds exceeding the personal stress average in 15-minute intervals).

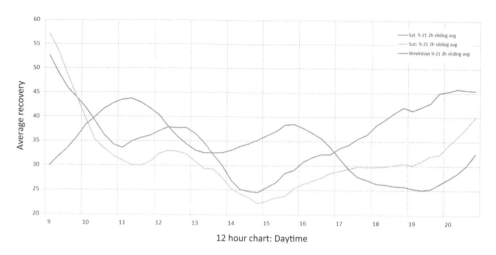

Figure 5. Recovery during the daytime (share of seconds exceeding the personal recovery average in 15-minute intervals).

Although our aim was not to study the data statistically or even to come up with generalisable conclusions, it is useful to examine individual differences in the observations. The greater the differences (deviation) between subjects, the more reason there is for us to believe that the observations are connected to individual factors. Looking at the figures for stress deviation (between subjects), night time appears to stand out especially clearly compared to daytime. Interestingly, in the small hours, around 4 am, the differences between the individual subjects' HRV are at their highest. In the so-called 'hour of the wolf' some of them are sound asleep, while others are apparently awake. The graph on daily deviations in recovery shows that the greatest individual differences are to be found during the daytime and even more so in the evenings.

The different profiles for stress and recovery raise the question of why deviance in stress among our test subjects is greatest at night time, while differences in recovery are greatest during the day. The additional observation that stress has a clear, collective, weekly and daily rhythm, which could not be seen as obviously in recovery, leads us to the main problem addressed by our research, that is, the social nature of the rhythms of everyday life. It appears that the stress rhythms are shaped by broader collective, social scheduling conventions concerning, for instance, sleeping times (see, e.g. European Commission, 2004). Could it be that stress (here measured in HRV) is connected more to the social practices shared by a large group of people (shopping times, times of physical activity etc.) while recovery is more dependent on individual resting habits, excluding sleeping times? If we had been studying entire families, it might have emerged that in families, too, the possibilities for recovery (e.g. naps) are socially determined.

When applying different methods of calculation, we came up with somewhat different results and interpretations. Overall, however, our data did show clear daily and weekly rhythms. In comparison to other weekdays, the stress and recovery profiles for both Saturdays and Sundays were unequivocal, as were the lowest recovery levels on Fridays. Nonetheless, it should be noted that some of our observations may be based on measuring mistakes in the gathering, calculation and interpretation of the data. For instance, we were unable to offer reasons for the stress peak on Saturday afternoon among the men.

We should also point out that we had largely to take the measures as given, and the patent-protected calculation algorithms were not made accessible to us, despite our requests. It is important in terms of a research design such as ours to take a critical view especially when it comes to the analysis of background factors, and perhaps see results mainly as a source of further questions. For example, why are the stress levels of physically active people lower during working hours? Could the answers lie in a strong sense of dignity that affects how people relate to disturbances in the daily rhythm, or in the effects of hard physical training on the functioning of the heart, nervous system and stress hormone?

Discussion

The 'social life of methods'

By iterating data consisting of millions of data points and applying many different calculation algorithms, we could conclude that alternative methods of representation, for example in the measurement intervals and scales, or different calculation approaches (standardising, aggregating, normalising) produced results that were open to interpretation, emphasising the heterogeneousness of both the data and the studied phenomenon. Mike Savage's recent discussion of the 'social life of methods' (2013) offers a reference point for our approach, as his article questioned research conventions and, for example, the strict distinction between qualitative and quantitative methods. Savage (2013, p. 18) emphasises a critical view of 'positivist practices' in empirical sociology, and is quite straightforward in suggesting that the decline of positivism can be seen in a critical attitude towards, for example, survey data and established statistical sampling methods.

Methodological experiments, politicisation of methods choices and an emphasis on historical specificity place importance on the continuously developing, interactive relationship between empiricism, theory and method, on the one hand, and varying ontological commitments on the other. In our case unstructured data led and forced us to continuously re-evaluate our thinking, and yet it is a question of more than a mere methodological transition or new track-and-trace technologies (e.g. DeLyser & Sui, 2012; Thrift, 2011). The conventions of presenting results, for example, are changing along with the emergence of real-time animation technologies. An experimental and innovative research orientation accepts inexact information; reality is always approached partially and imperfectly; and the results are often presented only in visual form instead of via statistical analysis (Simpson, 2012). In this perspective, the primary task of quantitative data is not to produce generalisable information on causal relations, but to place emphasis on the special nature of different phenomena and to reveal, for example, the mutual relations between various biological and social development trajectories that used to be regarded as isolated (e.g. Ruppert et al., 2013). This view also largely coincides with our perception of the significance of our research. The research design, which aimed at a descriptive analysis of collective rhythms, was critical with regards the research entity (to which we belonged) that emphasised a normative view of the health behaviour of individuals. In consequence of this, and as a result of the richness of measurements and data, we succeeded, to some extent, in deconstructing and reconstructing abstract and normative conceptions of stress and recovery, and also in questioning our own preconceptions concerning the value of established discourses of stress, recovery and rhythms of everyday life.

Frade (2013) has reasonably criticised the idea of sociologists 'getting their hands dirty' in new types of data and methodological plurality, noting that researchers are simultaneously taking part in the construction and renewal of a new kind of data-driven power-political agenda. We believe, however, that by collaborating in discussion among established sciences deploying new kinds of research designs one can also challenge dominant discourses and push for new interpretations. Our methodological experiments encourage participation in the diversification of means of measuring phenomena in everyday life by equally taking into account its conflicts, problems and silenced realities, including the problematic of recovery and rest. For instance, based on our participants' reflections, it emerged that subjective evaluation of stress differed from the data deduced from the heart. In this context, it is not possible to discuss the qualitative part of our research in more detail (Ruckenstein, 2014), but we offer few words about our findings in order to open them for further reflections.

How do the heart and mouth speak?

In the qualitative section of research, we identified periods among the test subjects which showed an exceptionally high level of stress or recovery, yet when we studied these moments, whether at work or at home, the heart-rate data and interview data sometimes produced conflicting information. In approximately every fifth identified incident, stress was revealed in talk but not by the heart. These situations were characterised by strong, culturally shared interpretations ('work stress') and strong emotions, such as recollections of personal relationships. In every tenth period under study, stress was expressed by the heart but not in talk. Activities typical of these periods involved transitions between work and leisure and different situations of preparation for upcoming events as well as consumption of alcohol.

Conflicts could also be observed in recovery. The periods where recovery was expressed in talk but not by the heart were characterised by the idea of 'forcing oneself to rest'. Every tenth period under study entailed this conflict. Those periods where recovery was expressed by the heart but not in talk were much more common. They were periods of, for example, routine activities like working at home or in the workplace and, generally, life devoid of surprises at large. Working life may perhaps be commonly experienced as more predictable than, for example, everyday life at home, which coincides with the viewpoint that underscores the 'minefield' of surprises and uncontrollability as a source of stress (Koolhaas et al., 2011). When we discussed these conflicted results with our subjects, they would occasionally offer their own perceptions of how they had found new worth for housework, including ironing or doing the dishes, because it was physiologically connected to recovery (Ruckenstein, 2014).

The results suggested that the heart recognises stress equally in daily life at home and in the workplace though, in public discussion, work stress receives much more attention than, for example, the everyday stress experienced by someone living alone or a stay-at-home parent. This is probably due to the dominance of economic talk in our society, which places more emphasis on the effective use of labour than on, say, good everyday life. Another observation we made with regards research could also be connected to this same phenomenon: research has paid little attention to recovery compared to stress. In both social research and in the physiological research of stress much more attention is given to the negative moments – stress, hurry and forced rhythm – than to moments of recovery and rest. In a similar vein, physiological research of stress has primarily focused on the attack-escape reactions of the autonomic (sympathetic) nervous system and other easily measurable activities. Much less interest has been given to the times, locations and practices of recovery and relaxation (Hinkle, 1974; Kugelman, 1992). This observation is all the more significant considering that stress is not life-threatening as such, whereas lack of recovery certainly is. Permanent deviations in bio-logical rhythms usually signify a pathological condition. Problems with sleep, for instance, are correlated with various health problems including diabetes, overweight or depression (Foster & Kreitzman, 2004; Koukkari & Sothern, 2006). For these reasons alone, the forced and unforced rhythms of daily lives merit more attention in sociological health research.

Our research suggests that measuring technologies, such as the HRV device, can not only overcome problems connected with observing activities, but also with inactivities; for example, bodily movement could offer a new way of identifying 'passivities' (Löfgren & Ehn, 2010) and overcoming the difficult problem of how questions of 'passive activity' are articulated. This could promote new kinds of research designs in the field of health and medicine where activities such as watching TV are typically per-ceived purely and solely as something negative, correlating to lifestyle diseases (Pantzar, 2010).

What can we learn from rhythms of everyday life?

Biotemporal rhythms and especially variations within a day are a consequence of the network-like structure of the human body and nervous system. In the past, sociological time-use research has been more interested in socio-temporal rhythms (and cycles) which also often involve complex feedbacks (e.g. Zerubavel, 1981); along with new body monitors, however, novel hybrid disciplines can emerge, such as chronobiology, that integrate the empirical research of bio- and socio-temporal rhythms. Chronobiology has identified a large number of biotemporal rhythms in animals (including humans), from microscopically short cycles to those that extend over the entire lifespan (e.g. Foster & Kreitzman, 2004; Koukkari & Sothern, 2006), often with different hormonal (bio-temporal) feedbacks to be found in the background. For example, with human beings the levels of the so-called stress hormone, cortisol, vary within the day, reaching their highest in the morning and becoming increasingly lower in the course of the day (Semmer et al., 2004). Rhythms of stress and recovery can therefore be seen as products of the coupled effect of human physiology and cultural processes.

It is also known from time-use sociology that conflicted expectations and the need to 'juggle' different rhythms of everyday life seem to increase an individual's experience of stress (e.g. Southerton, 2006). Such critical moments could consist, for example, in prepar-ing for a vacation or a party. In a study carried out by Southerton (2003) based on inter-view data, times in a person's life appear to be experientially divided into 'red moments of stress' and 'blue moments of recovery'. In this example, the red moments are linked with preparing for events such as the weekend, a work trip or Christmas, while the blue moments represent the pleasure of enjoying the fruit of preparations.

Focusing on the physiology of the heart offers a clear contrast to the sociology of everyday life, where the phenomenological or constructivist aspects have had a prominent role. Contrary to the views propounded by many theorists of everyday life (e.g. Gouldner, 1975), the heart does not make a distinction between, say, a 'disalienated' lifeworld and 'official' systems (for the distinction, see Highmore, 2002). A notable conflict that we came across in our research was that the heart (body) and mouths (culture) of our test subjects were not always 'speaking the same language'. In other words, HRV and subjective interpretations of stress were sending mutually contradictory messages. For this reason alone, it would be useful for social scientists to become better acquainted with human biology, and medical doctors with the social sphere.

In the future, combining, for example, time-use research and 'cardiograms' might produce a whole new kind of insight into the conditions and consequences of human everyday activity. Tools that have initially been developed for professional use will establish themselves as a natural part of individuals' everyday life and self-monitoring practices (Pantzar & Ruckenstein, 2014; Ruckenstein & Pantzar, 2015). This means, on the one hand, that medical interpretation and vocabulary will gradually approach the sphere of 'ordinary people' (Beaudin, Intille, & Morris, 2006), while, on the other, 'personalised medicine' (Swan, 2013) will present its own challenges to the medical profession, as people become 'lay experts' on health conditions. Closely corresponding with this, the scope and focus of methods used in social research should also be widened.

Conclusions

With our research project, with its aim of describing and visualising the rhythmic movements of stress and recovery, we wish to contribute to a wider biopolitical endeavour and a turn towards New Materialism to recognise the social dimension and performance of the human body, especially the heart. Our study forced us to evaluate measuring practices and the value of digital data from multiple perspectives. The quantitative and qualitative results supported each other to a certain extent, while also splitting out in different directions.

The quantitative results offer a new kind of access to human life, continuing the history of conquering unknown regions by opening the pulse of human physiology, in this case the heartbeat, for inspection (Haraway, 1998). As a practice, this type of measurement means chopping and breaking everyday life into parts, rendering particular slices of human life visible, and thus requiring us to take a stance on them. This approach to measuring is also an intervention, because it produces information by sketching out unforeseen dimensions. However, instead of pursuing the goals of universal applicability or reproducibility, our research design strove to reveal the conditions of research of this type, paying attention to what they restrict and enable.

With such a difficult, challenging and laborious research project the learning curve was considerable. Inspired by the discussions that have been raised by the approach outlined in Savage's article on the social life of methods (2013), we want to underline how by 'getting one's hands dirty' one can critically assess the established and rigidified epistemological and ontological commitments linked to health research. We also discovered how methods constrain research participation: some people are eager to quantify their existence by even the most peculiar and strenuous means, while others would under no circumstances subject themselves to measurement of their everyday, intimate lives.

When we started our study the hypothesis was that the human heart beats not only as a part of the human nervous system but also as a part of human social life. We ventured to study social rhythms by using body monitors developed in the field of sport physiology, having to take a lot as given, both when it came to measuring technology and interpretation of the calculation algorithms. Despite different methods of calculation and failures therein, our initial perception was confirmed as the research project proceeded. Recognising the connection between the cyclical processes in the human body and states of balance or imbalance in the metabolism or heart beat can be problematic in science in terms of a division of labour. In highly simplified terms, the 'autonomic' or 'sympathetic' nervous systems have not been a matter of concern for social scientists any more than the causes of daily stress have been for the medical profession. Yet, human biology has come to the fore in recent years in the social sciences along with developments in medical science and new theories on corporeality (Coole & Frost, 2010; Freese, Li, & Wade, 2003; Rose, 2013). The development of data and storing technologies has, and will continue to have, an essential impact on this development. What is happening is not merely a question of a 'sensory revolution' (Swan, 2012) or a new 'age of data' (Bowker, Baker, Millerand, & Ribes, 2010) but of a more profound change which will hopefully find a more solid place for the human body and nature in the social sciences. The essential thing is to recognise not only the opportunities provided by new mobile and digital instruments but also the preconditions they entail. For social scientists, this calls for a curious and unprejudiced attitude and a commitment to becoming involved with and affected by new types of data and research methods.

Note

1. The HRV monitor (electrodes) was attached directly to participants' chests at two points: the device needs to be removed only during water sports and when showering.

Disclosure statement

No potential conflict of interest was reported by the authors.

References

Acharya, U. R., Joseph, K. P., Kannathal, N., Lim, C. M., & Suri, J. S. (2006). Heart rate variability: A review. *Medical and Biological Engineering and Computing, 44*, 1031–1051. doi:10.1007/s11517-006-0119-0

Andersson, K., Nafus, D., Rattenbury, T., & Aipperspach, R. (2009). Numbers have qualities too: Experiences with ethno-mining. *EPIC Proceedings 2009, 1*, 123–140. doi:10.1111/j.1559-8918.2009.tb00133.x

Beaudin, J., Intille, S., & Morris, M. (2006). To track or not to track: User reactions to concepts in longitudinal health monitoring. *Journal of Medical Internet Research, 8*(4), e29. doi:10.2196/jmir.8.4.e29.

Bender, J., & Marinar, M. (2010). *The culture of diagram*. Stanford, CA: Stanford University Press.

Bowker, G., Baker, K., Millerand, F., & Ribes, D. (2010). Toward information infrastructure studies: Ways of knowing in a networked environment. In J. Hunsinger, L. Klastrup, & M. Allen (Eds.), *International handbook of internet research* (pp. 97–117). Dordrecht: Springer.

Coole, D., & Frost, S. (Eds.). (2010). *New materialisms: Ontology, agency, and politics*. Durham: Duke University Press.

DeLyser, D., & Sui, D. (2012). Crossing the qualitative-quantitative divide II: Inventive approaches to big data, mobile methods, and rhythmanalysis. *Progress in Human Geography, 37*, 293–305. doi:10.1177/0309132512444063

Edwards, J., Harvey, P., & Wade, P. (Eds.). (2010). *Technologized images, technologized bodies*. New York, NY: Berghahn Books.

Ellegård, K., & Vilhelmson, B. (2004). Home as a pocket of local order: Everyday activities and the friction of distance. *Geografiska Annaler: Series B, Human Geography, 86*, 281–296. doi:10.1111/j.0435-3684.2004.00168.x

European Commission. (2004). *How Europeans spend their time. Everyday life of women and men. Data 1998–2002. Eurostat. Pocketbooks: Theme 3: Population and social conditions*. Luxembourg: Office for Official Publications of the European Communities.

Foster, R., & Kreitzman, L. (2004). *Rhythms of life: The biological clocks that control the daily lives of every living things*. New Haven: Yale University Press.

Frade, C. (2013). *Time and method: After survival, for a renewed praxis of social theory* (CRESC Working Paper Series, 132, pp. 1–17). University of Manchester. Retrieved from http://usir.salford.ac.uk/id/eprint/30630

Freese, J., Li, J.-C., & Wade, L. (2003). The potential relevances of biology to social inquiry. *Annual Review of Sociology, 29*, 233–256. doi:10.1146/annurev.soc.29.010202.100012

Gershuny, J. (2000). *Changing times. Work and leisure in postindustrial society*. Oxford: Oxford University Press.

Gouldner, A. (1975). Sociology and the everyday life. In L. Corer (Ed.), *The idea of social structure, papers in honor of Robert K. Merton* (pp. 417–432). New York, NY: Harcourt Brace Jovanovich.

Haraway, D. (1998). Deanimations: Maps and portraits of life itself. In P. Galison & C. Jones (Eds.), *Picturing science, producing Art* (pp. 181–210). New York, NY: Routledge.

Heaphy, E., & Dutton, J. (2008). Positive social interactions and human body at work: Linking organizations and physiology. *Academy of Management Review, 33*, 137–162. doi:10.5465/AMR.2008.27749365

Highmore, B. (2002). *Everyday life and cultural theory*. London: Routledge.

Hinkle, L. E. (1974). The concept of "stress" in the biological and social sciences. *International Journal of Psychiatry in Medicine, 5*, 335–357. doi:10.2190/91DK-NKAD-1XP0-Y4RG

Kettunen, J. (1999). *Methodological and empirical advances in the quantitative analysis of spontaneous responses in psychophysiological time series*. Helsinki: Helsingin yliopiston psykologian laitoksen tutkimuksia no. 21. Retrieved from http://urn.fi/URN:ISBN:951-45-8719-7

Koolhaas, J., Bartolomucci, A., Buwalda, B., de Boer, S. F., Flügge, G., Korte, S. M., … Fuchs, E. (2011). Stress revisited: A critical evaluation of the stress concept. *Neuroscience and Biobehavioral Reviews, 35*, 1291–301. doi:10.1016/j.neubiorev.2011.02.003

Koukkari, W., & Sothern, R. (2006). *Introducing biological rhythms*. New York, NY: Springer.

Kugelman, R. (1992). *Stress. The nature and history of engineered grief*. London: Praeger.

Lefebvre, H. (1992/2004). *Rhythmanalysis: Space, time and everyday life*. Athlone, Contemporary European Thinkers. London: Continuum.

Löfgren, O., & Ehn, B. (2010). *The secret world of doing nothing*. Berkeley: University of California Press.

Lupton, D. (2012). M-health and health promotion: The digital cyborg and surveillance society. *Social Theory & Health, 10*, 229–244. doi:10.1057/sth.2012.6

Lupton, D. (2015, September 27). *Lively data, social fitness and biovalue: The intersections of health self-tracking and social media*. Available at SSRN: http://ssrn.com/abstract=2666324

Michelson, W. (2005). *Time use. Expanding the explanatory power of the social sciences*. London: Paradigm Publisher.

Pantzar, M. (2010). Future shock – Discussing changing temporal architecture of daily life. *Journal of Future Studies, 14*(4), 1–22.

Pantzar, M., & Ruckenstein, M. (2014). The heart of everyday analytics: Identifying practices and future domains in self-tracking. *Consumption Markets & Culture.* doi:10.1080/10253866.2014.899213

Pantzar, M., & Shove, E. (2010). Time in practice – Discussing rhythms of practice complexes. Ethnologia Europaea. *Journal of European Ethnology, 40*(1), 19–29.

Rosa, H. (2003). Social acceleration: Ethical and political consequences of a desynchronized high-speed society. *Constellations, 10*, 3–33. doi:10.1111/1467-8675.00309

Rose, N. (2013). The human sciences in a biological age. *Theory, Culture and Society, 30*(1), 3–34. doi:10.1177/0263276412456569

Ruckenstein, M. (2013). Temporalities of addiction. In L. Hansson, U. Holmberg & H. Brembeck (Eds.), *Making sense of consumption. Selections from the 2nd nordic conference on consumer research 2012* (pp. 107–118). Göteborg: University of Gothenburg.

Ruckenstein, M. (2014). Visualized and interacted life: Personal analytics and engagements with data doubles. *Societies, 4*(1), 68–84.

Ruckenstein, M., & Pantzar, M. (2015). Beyond the quantified self: Thematic exploration of a dataistic paradigm. *New Media & Society.* doi:10.1177/1461444815609081

Ruppert, E., Law, J., & Savage, M. (2013). Reassembling social science methods: The challenge of digital devices. *Theory, Culture & Society, 30*(4), 22–46. doi:10.1177/0263276413484941

Savage, M. (2013). The 'social life of methods': A critical introduction. *Theory, Culture & Society, 30* (4), 3–21. doi:10.1177/0263276413486160

Schatzki, T. (2010). *Timespace and human activity.* Lanham, MD: Lexington Books.

Selye, H. (1973). The evolution of stress concept. *American Scientist, 61*, 692–699. Retrieved from http://www.jstor.org/stable/27844072

Semmer, N., Grebner, S., & Elfering, A. (2004). Beyond self-report: Using observational, physiological and situation-based measures in research on occupational stress. In P. Perrewé & D. Ganster (Eds.), *Emotional and physiological processes and positive intervention strategies* (pp. 205–263). Amsterdam: Elsevier.

Simpson, P. (2012). Apprehending everyday rhythms: Rhythmanalysis, time-lapse photography, and the space-times of street performance. *Cultural Geographies, 19*, 423–445. doi:10.1177/1474474012443201

Southerton, D. (2003). "Squeezing time": Allocating practices, co-ordinating networks and scheduling society. *Time & Society, 12*, 5–25. doi:10.1177/0961463X03012001001

Southerton, D. (2006). Analysing the temporal organization of daily life: Social constraints, practices and their allocation. *Sociology, 40*, 435–454. doi:10.1177/0038038506063668

Swan, M. (2012). Sensor mania! The internet of things, objective metrics, and the quantified self 2.0. *Journal of Sensor and Actuator Network, 1*, 217–253. doi:10.3390/jsan1030217

Swan, M. (2013). The Quantified Self: Fundamental disruption in big data science and biological discovery. *Big Data, 1*, 85–99. doi:10.1089/big.2012.0002

Thompson, E. (1967). Time, work-discipline, and industrial capitalism. *Past and Present, A Journal of Historical Studies, 38*(1), 56–97. Retrieved from http://www.jstor.org/stable/649749

Thrift, N. (2011). Lifeworld Inc. – And what to do about it. *Environment and Planning D: Society and Space, 29*, 5–26. doi:10.1068/d0310

Uusitalo, A., Mets, T., Martinmäki, K., Mauno, S., Kinnunen, U., & Rusko, H. (2011). Heart rate variability related to effort at work. *Applied Ergonomics, 42*, 830–838. doi:10.1016/j.apergo.2011.01.005

Zerubavel, E. (1981). *Hidden rhythms: Schedules and calendars in social life.* Berkeley: University of California Press.

Clinical self-tracking and monitoring technologies: negotiations in the ICT-mediated patient–provider relationship

Enrico Maria Piras and Francesco Miele

ABSTRACT

This paper discusses mediation in the patient–provider relationship arising from the introduction of digital technology for a specific form of monitoring: 'clinical self-tracking'. Focusing on the management of type 1 diabetes, a condition that requires significant self-management by patients, we describe how the actors negotiated a new ICT-mediated relationship in three hospital departments. The analysis followed a qualitative design and was carried out by interviewing patients, clinicians and technology developers and by analysing messages exchanged through the ICT tool. We first show how each department customised the system by drawing on already existing care practices, organisational goals and representations of the department's desired relationship with the patients. We then focus on patient–provider relationships, showing that, while the clinical self-tracking sometimes followed the path desired by the providers, at other times, it developed in unexpected ways. We distinguish among three emerging categories of self-tracking: self-tracking for remote management, self-tracking for e-learning and self-tracking as boundary setting. The analysis reveals how the new patient–provider relationship arises from an open-ended process. Providers can push self-tracking practices but cannot steer them; and patients, through an unexpected use of the self-tracking technologies, are able to negotiate a desired relationship with providers.

Introduction

Health self-tracking has become a popular research issue in recent years. This interest is due to a number of partially related causes, such as the increase in people with long-term health conditions, the growing importance of self-care, the spread of miniaturised and easy-to-use measuring devices and smartphone applications and the availability of social networking platforms. With some basic computer skills and some low-cost gadgets, it is relatively easy to produce and share an amount of personal health information unimaginable only a few years ago.

The new technologies have been hailed by healthcare managers and policy-makers as offering opportunities to reshape the healthcare system. Groups of tech-enthusiasts have played a significant role in raising awareness about the potential of self-tracking modalities. The Quantified Self movement (http://quantifiedself.com) has established itself as a new approach in which the ability of laypeople to collect and interpret data enables them to find patterns and improve their quality of life (Li, Dey, & Forlizzi, 2010). While there is still little evidence of health benefits associated with Quantified Self practices (Ledger & McCaffrey, 2014), some studies have focused on the surveillance and control aspects of self-tracking (Allen, 2008; Bossewitch & Sinnreich, 2013) and resistance practices enacted by users (Fox, 2015). Moreover, the demographic categories that could benefit most from Quantified Self practices – such as elderly people with chronic conditions – are not a target market for the companies producing these technologies (Doyle, Walsh, Sassu, & McDonagh, 2014). These results leave open the question of whether self-tracking practices contribute to exacerbating the differences among social groups in their access to new health services.

Most of the debate on health self-tracking seems to be modelled on a script in which two irreconcilable positions can be easily discerned. On the one hand, there are the techno-enthusiasts who consider self-tracking technologies and practices to be a turning point in health management (Rivera-Pelayo, Zacharias, Müller, & Braun, 2012; Swan, 2012); on the other, there are those who see them as embodiments of a corporate and public health agenda that will eventually lead to the medicalisation of society (Conrad, 2007) and which must be resisted through subversive practices (Fox, 2015).

This polarisation does not do justice to the rich phenomenology of health self-tracking, instead reducing it to a confrontation between 'nightmare' scenarios and those full of 'promise' (Pols, 2012). This contrast is a recurrent trope in debates on new technologically propelled changes. The techno-utopian scenarios presented by both academia and policy-makers need to be challenged (see Lupton, 2014a, 2016), and there is a need for critical analysis of self-tracking practices and how they relate to the ongoing transformation of health care.

For these purposes, it is necessary to shift the focus from the future to the present, considering the social practices of self-tracking and the place that they occupy in people's everyday lives. Interesting in this regard is the classification by Lupton (2014b) of the different ways in which trackers organize, analyse and interpret data. Lupton identifies five categories of self-tracking: private, communal, pushed, imposed and exploited (Lupton, 2014b). Thus, how one keeps track of one's diet differs according to whether the data are collected for oneself (private self-tracking), shared with an online community of people who want to lose weight (communal self-tracking), collected on a doctor's advice (pushed self-tracking), required by an employer (imposed self-tracking) or given to a company that wants to profile its customers (exploited self-tracking). This classification has, among other things, the merit of showing how the Quantified Self movement – which has, in some ways, 'cannibalised' the debate on self-tracking – constitutes only two of the components of the phenomenon (i.e. private and communal self-tracking). In the other cases, tracking is part of an asymmetric relationship between the tracker and the organisations that push, impose or exploit the tracking itself.

In this study, we focus on 'pushed self-tracking', which refers to practices initiated in response to external encouragement rather than those that are self-generated and private. This mode of self-tracking is common in the healthcare sector, where providers persuade patients to keep track of certain health-related information.

We are interested in documenting the mediations in the patient–provider relationship arising from the redistribution in the care network of long-established disease management tasks made possible by the use of digital technologies. We report an empirically grounded analysis of the transformation of already established self-tracking practices in the management of type 1 diabetes, a chronic condition that requires significant effort by patients in self-care practices. The study follows the process of introducing a digital platform that allows patients to keep track of their health data and allows providers to access them in real time, and it describes how the actors negotiate a new relationship through its use.

The paper is structured as follows. In the next section, we introduce the notion of 'clinical self-tracking', a social practice shared by patients and clinicians. The findings, preceded by the methodological section, are organised into two sub-sections. We first present how the clinicians customised the platform to gain more direct supervision of patients. We then show the clinical self-tracking practices and three different forms of appropriation of the platform by patients and providers. We conclude by discussing how self-tracking can mediate quite different patient–provider relationships.

Clinical self-tracking and monitoring technologies

Clinical self-tracking is a part of a larger set of social practices regarding personal health information management that has been recently investigated (Ancker et al., 2015; Moen & Brennan, 2005; Piras & Zanutto, 2010). While 'personal health information management' often refers to the management of institutional documents, 'self-tracking' specifically denotes the monitoring of data that can only be collected by patients themselves – sometimes also referred to as 'observation of daily living' (Brennan & Casper, 2015).

In the management of chronic conditions, delegation of parameter measurements to patients or caregivers is a part of a therapeutic alliance in which data are used by patients for self-management purposes but are also shared with care providers. We shall refer to this as 'clinical self-tracking', a practice that is often part of a family of 'self-actions' that patients can be required to perform (e.g. self-measuring, self-administering and self-dosing) to improve independent management of their condition. Self-tracking may play a fundamental role in the patient–provider relationship; indeed, in some cases, it is the actual cornerstone of the relationship.

Clinical self-tracking practices have certain characteristics that we shall illustrate with specific reference to type 1 diabetes.

Practices are pushed by healthcare providers. Self-tracking practices are initiated following providers' advice for either diagnostic or therapeutic purposes (MacLeod, Tang, & Carpendale, 2013). In some cases, the analysis of self-tracked data is the objective of the patient–provider encounter itself, and providers may refuse to examine patients who do not perform the self-tracking activities required.

Tracking requires education. Providers use training to educate patients on tracking (Funnell & Anderson, 2004). Even seemingly simple tracking activities require instruction (e.g. measuring weight). More complex activities require providers to instruct patients on the use of a given instrument (e.g. a glucose meter) and to educate them on how to interpret the results (e.g. to identify an alert indicating hypoglycaemia). Education can even be delegated to different providers, with doctors usually providing the 'theory' and others, the 'techniques'.

Data are standardised. Doctors require patients to collect data uniformly over time, and they provide tracking tools that help in this regard (e.g. logbooks). The standardisation helps providers and users in their analysis of the data. Data gathering is generally framed in a predefined scheme of interpretation: self-tracking is less an activity aimed at discovering new relations among data than an activity based on codified medical knowledge where associations among data are already established.

Analysis of data is performed also by patients, and it leads to action. Whilst traditional health data analysis is performed only by providers, in clinical self-tracking, patients are required to have interpretation skills (Piras & Zanutto, 2014). They are required to understand what they track, and they are instructed on how to react appropriately (e.g. by modifying the therapy or by calling the doctor).

Tracking has a situated meaning. The specific sense of clinical self-tracking must be considered in the context of the organisational practices of which it is part (Gherardi, 2010; Oudshoorn, 2012). The same self-tracking activities may be performed to delegate an active role to patients, to monitor their compliance, to educate newly diagnosed patients or to delegate most of the care to patients themselves.

Tracking evolves over time and leads to different configurations of the patient–provider relationship. Over time, patients may perform self-tracking differently (e.g. tracking new parameters, using different tracking tools) and gain an understanding of their condition which is more accurate than that of their providers. This may give rise to new forms of therapeutic alliance in which patients and providers are both considered 'experts' (Piras & Zanutto, 2014).

In numerous clinical settings, patients are required to keep track of parameters for various purposes (e.g. management, diagnosis) and which carry various levels of complexity. For purely illustrative purposes, we can imagine arranging clinical self-tracking activities along two Cartesian axes, one representing the amount of information to be collected and the other representing the amount of learning required, including new concepts, procedures and techniques. We thus can divide self-tracking activities into those that require few data and little learning (e.g. monitoring the body weight of a patient with chronic heart failure), numerous data and little learning (e.g. a food logbook for an obese patients), few data but high learning (e.g. a logbook of peritoneal dialysis) and numerous data and high learning (e.g. management of type 1 diabetes).

Type 1 diabetes is a metabolic disorder characterised by instability of glycaemia in the blood caused by the destruction of the pancreatic cells. This results in a deficit of insulin, which must be corrected by injecting synthetic insulin. The management of diabetes is based on the patients' self-assessment of their state of health several times a day with the consequent insulin correction (Funnell & Anderson, 2004). This model has been made possible by the increasing availability of patient-controlled technologies for diabetes self-management (e.g. glucometers, urine ketones testing kits) and for insulin self-dosage (e.g. syringes, pens and pumps). In this pathology, self-tracking is performed intensively: patients track a large amount of data, analyse them together with doctors and engage in a continuous learning process. This makes diabetes an excellent case for the study of clinical self-tracking.

Methodology

The research project reported here flanked a clinical trial aimed at quantifying the effectiveness and the acceptability of a self-tracking/remote-monitoring platform for type 1 diabetes patients. A smartphone application enabled patients to keep track of all the information relative to their diabetes (e.g. measurements, therapy, symptoms and diet); it also included functions to support decision-making (i.e. a carbohydrate count feature, a bolus calculator, graphs and trend-tracking indexes). The web-based dashboard accessible by doctors was endowed with a system of rule-based alarms designed to send an alert to clinicians and/or patients in the presence of certain data or combinations of data. Moreover, the platform had an inbuilt messaging system that worked as a secure email service between patients and providers.

The trial lasted three months and involved three hospital departments of a mountainous Italian region. Each department specialised in diabetes care. Each department focused on a particular patient profile and enrolled 10–15 patients. 'Paediatrics' selected children and adolescents with either poorly controlled diabetes, a recent diagnosis or who used an insulin pump. 'DC-Adult' focused on people with poorly controlled diabetes. 'DC-Pregnant' selected pregnant women; women with gestational diabetes were excluded on the basis that they did not have any previous experience with management of the disease. These choices targeted patient profiles that, according to physicians, would benefit from the stricter monitoring and the frequent reminders about correct disease management that the platform could provide.

The project presented here was based on qualitative research conducted alongside the clinical trial. We focused on the self-tracking practices of patients, the changes in organisational practices due to the introduction of the new technology in the departments and, finally, the changes in the patient–provider relationship. Close attention was paid to the forms of appropriation of self-tracking and monitoring technologies by both providers and patients and the meaning of health information management in each context.

The study was conducted by means of semi-structured interviews with patients (at the conclusion of the clinical trial), caregivers, healthcare professionals and the developers of the technologies (see Table 1). Patients and parents were interviewed on self-tracking practices and changes in their relationships with the clinicians. The developers were interviewed to understand the logic behind the development of the system and its adaptations in each department (see Table 2). All of the healthcare professionals involved in the clinical trial (i.e. those using the system) were interviewed to obtain information about the adaptations required and the new relationship established with the patients. The number of interviewees varied according to the specific organisation of each department.[1] The adult diabetic patients were interviewed on their own; in the cases of children and teenagers, one or both of the parents were also involved (four interviews); for the youngest ones (eight interviews), only the parents were interviewed.

Patients and their relatives were interviewed at home. Written consent was obtained; this form was among the documents signed upon enrolment for the clinical trial. Interviews lasted 45–60 minutes, and they were transcribed verbatim. The patient–provider relationship was further explored through the analysis of free-text messages exchanged between patients/caregivers and doctors via the system. The messages concerned analysis of patients' data, inquiries and comments on insulin therapy, diet and the self-management of diabetes.

Table 1. Targets involved and fieldwork.

Department	Subjects	Interviews
Paediatric unit (Paediatrics)	Children/adolescents with either: • a recent onset of disease • poorly controlled diabetes • an insulin pump	Eight parents, four patients + parents, one medical doctor
Diabetes Centre 1 (DC-adults)	Adults (aged) with: • poorly controlled diabetes	Eight patients, two medical doctors, one diabetes nurse
Diabetes Centre 2 (DC-pregnant)	Pregnant women with: • high-intensity insulin treatment	Nine patients, one medical doctor, one diabetes nurse
Research Centre	Developing team	One project manager, one computer scientists, one developer

All of the empirical materials (e.g. interviews, messages) were coded using template analysis (King, 1998). Preliminary labels based on the interview outline were used to segment the text. The work on the text guided the analysis and led to refinement of the labels and the creation of new ones. The themes that guided construction of the template originated from the dimensions addressed by the interview outline:

- division of labour between patients/parents and healthcare providers;
- self-tracking and everyday life;
- effect of real-time information-sharing on the patient–provider relationship.

Table 2. Topics of interview.

	Patients and caregivers	Healthcare professionals	Developers
Patient–provider relationship (before digital self-tracking)	• Education at onset • Self-management and self-tracking practices • Use of self-tracked data	• Education at onset • Education during clinical encounters • Use of patient-tracked data	Not applicable
Customisation of self-tracking platform	Not applicable	• Activation of additional functions • Configuration of the rule-based alarms	• Activation of additional functions • Configuration of the rule-based alarms
Use of self-tracking platform	• Self-tracking practices (collection and data analysis); • Relation between self-tracking and other care practices • Changes in patient–provider relationship	• Use of patient-tracked data (analysis) • Relation between analysis of patient-tracked data and other organisational practices • Changes in patient–provider relationship	Not applicable

Findings

We shall organize this section into two parts. First, we describe how the technology was customised by each department before the beginning of the trial. Second, we analyse the emergent use and reconfiguration of the patient–provider relationship.

Organisational customisation

Before the trial started, each department was given the opportunity to customize the system.

Already-existing care practices, organisational goals and representations of the desired new relationship with the patients contributed to reshaping the technology. Doctors suggested customisations that could either strengthen already-existing relationships or redefine them. When patients' education was considered the focus of the patient–doctor relationship, the system was customised to increase the autonomy of patients; when professionals were mainly concerned about patients' compliance with their prescriptions, the system became a way to control and enforce patients' care practices. The modifications allowed were the activation/deactivation of some additional functions in the electronic logbook used by patients and configuration of the rule-based alarms.

The paediatric department (Paediatrics) and the Diabetes Centre 1 (DC-Adults) selected an identical configuration. They requested activation of all the additional functions on the patients' apps, and they decided that alarms should be received by both the department and the patients. More precisely, they decided that six alarms regarding everyday management should be received by both patients and the department; two alarms regarding hypoglycaemia and hyperglycaemia trends should be received by the patients only; one alarm regarding risk should be received by the department only.

These choices were consistent with the aims of the experimental scheme: to support patients in self-monitoring and increase the autonomy of patients and their caregivers in decision-making while allowing medical intervention in emergencies. Despite the similarities, however, Paediatrics and DC-Adults had quite different understandings of what the system meant. Paediatrics heavily relied on empowerment and was confident that patients would be able to recognize abnormal values–trends and to understand autonomously whether their estimates of food and insulin therapy intake were accurate. Despite the faith in patient education, Paediatrics considered the system as a means to monitor non-adherence.

> Probably at times when you get worse, you're more motivated to do things […]. So patients with poor compliance but who don't want to be supervised are the ones that we want to monitor. (Paediatrics, physician)

DC-Adults showed less confidence than the other departments in the capability of their patients to make good choices and invited them to use the functions (such as the carbohydrate calculator) to receive advice.

> If you tell the program how much food you're eating, how many carbohydrates, it translates that information into insulin and tells you 'do this amount of insulin'. You may not do it, or decide to do a different amount, but it gives you an input or datum to think about. (DC-Adults, head of department).

DC-Pregnant customised the system in a radically different way. Pregnancy alters the patient–provider relationship, leading to strict surveillance. Mismanagement of blood glucose can have strong consequences for the foetus, putting the pregnancy itself at risk. In the department in question, for instance, a diabetic woman who ordinarily had two or three examinations a year would have one every two weeks during pregnancy. The system was conceived by the department as a tool that allowed even stricter monitoring. It was also decided that the additional functions should not be allowed because they might lead to autonomous decision-making; instead, the department preferred to provide strict recommendations. The doctors also decided that all alarms but two would be set exclusively for them. Whilst self-management was foregrounded by providers in Paediatrics and DC-Adults, for DC-Pregnant, the technology was a means to receive information in real time from the patient, enabling providers to make their own interpretations and provide therapeutic prescriptions.

> Our alarms are only seen by the doctor and not by the patient … this is because we're dealing with a pregnant woman, and in a very fragile period of life from a psychological point of view, who is already very involved because she also has diabetes, and of course her goal is to have a normal child, a normal pregnancy … therefore, the fewer problems we impose on the woman, the better. (DC-Pregnant, head of department)

The different customisations can be interpreted as different ways to inscribe, in the technical artefact, a distinctive meaning of the self-tracking practices to be performed by the patient. Paediatrics considered self-tracking to be an autonomous endeavour, and it saw the system as a tool with which to obtain a second opinion and monitor the patients' behaviour. A similar view was taken by DC-adults, though in this case the system was regarded as a guiding tool in self-managing practices. DC-pregnant, however, considered self-tracking to be merely a practice with which to receive information and provide recommendations. The different positions of the three clinical centres can be summarised by the following interview excerpt, where a technician in charge of customising the system talks about choices concerning additional features.

> It depends on the view of the doctors. The ambition of [Paediatrics] was that the calculation of bolus would educate the patients into comparing their abilities with those of the system. So it's a form of tutoring. [DC-Adults] deals with patients who have little familiarity with calculating the bolus and the carbohydrates. It emerged from discussion with the chief consultant that he wanted the patient to avoid making mistakes. He saw it as a function that the patient calculated and accepted. [DC-Pregnant] did not want it. (Design team, technician)

Emerging patient–provider relationships

While the goal of the clinical trial was to assess the usability and perceived value of the system, both providers and patients had little to say about the technology itself. Apart from some minor comments, every user was satisfied and quickly learned to use the system. The different ways in which patients used the technology can be explained by considering their choices as reactions to the modification of the patient–provider relationship triggered by the system's introduction into the already-existing self-tracking practices. These patterns show that clinical self-tracking at times followed the path desired by providers, while at others, it developed in unexpected ways, betraying the doctors' expectations. We distinguish among three non-exclusive categories:

(1) *Self-tracking for remote management:* performed so that providers can make decisions, while patients have limited, if any, power for autonomous decision-making. Pregnant women and caregivers of children with a recent diabetes onset fall into this category.

(2) *Self-tracking for e-learning:* performed to receive education both from the system and online from providers. Most adult patients fall into this category.

(3) *Self-tracking as boundary setting:* performed for self-management purposes; data are not shared with providers, reaffirming the patient's independence from providers in disease management. Young and adult patients with poorly controlled diabetes use the technology in this way.

Self-tracking for remote management

The high number of choices to be constantly made requires patients to be able to interpret data and take autonomous decisions. For limited periods of time, however, patients can be considered fragile and in need of assistance from doctors. Hospitalisation, pregnancy, a recent onset of diabetes or the first months of using an insulin pump are good examples of short-term conditions that are managed by increasing patient–provider communication and face-to-face encounters.

DC-Pregnant was the one that most forcefully interpreted the system as a tool with which to redefine the doctor–patient relationship by making it more prescriptive. Pregnant women with diabetes must monitor their blood sugar values with particular care because poor control of glucose levels can endanger pregnancy, and prolonged hyperglycaemia induces the foetus to produce a massive amount of the hormone insulin with consequent abnormal growth.

> We've seen your Friday glucose readings. I'd say they are not in the desired range; we'd like to understand what happened. You didn't input the dinner composition, and the pre-dinner insulin is missing: did you do it? The post-dinner reading is low: why didn't you eat? Please try to be more accurate if you can. (DC-Pregnant, message from doctor to patient)

The system is meant to control the patient's status in real time. She, in turn, is regarded as a data provider with little or no autonomy. This is a major shift in the relationship with the diabetic centre, which is mostly accepted by patients who consider themselves not fully able to manage the new condition.

> [With the system] I feel safer, I think, because I know that everyone sees how my blood sugar levels are going and can change the therapy [...] [So] for me, it's more convenient [...] if I had to come here every two weeks it'd be a hassle because I live some distance away. (DC-Pregnant, interview with a pregnant woman, 39 years old)

In this manner, moreover, the frequency of face-to-face encounters is reduced because the system allows for constant monitoring. For some patients, especially pregnant women living far from the hospital and in the last months before delivery, the transformation of some examinations into teleconsultations is a boon.

However, even if we restrict the analysis to the patients who accepted the transformation of their relationship with providers, we find evidence of fatigue and tensions within the care team. Despite being recognised as useful, the strict monitoring was regarded as interrupting a normal relationship that those patients wanted to re-establish with the provider after the pregnancy.

> No ... now you do it because you have a goal [that] you care about. Now, you're always supervised, but after [delivery], it would be like being really sick. (DC-Pregnant, response of a pregnant woman (33 years old) when asked about using the system after delivery)

Even if they believed that stricter monitoring was necessary, patients could sometimes elude, partially or totally, the doctor's prescriptions. The latter were sometimes perceived as excessively rigid and uncaring about food tastes, lifestyle and physical characteristics. In these cases, after patients received the doctor's interpretations, they made their own interpretations of the tracked data: interpretations compatible with their care needs and, at the same time, adequate to maintain glucose levels within the desired range.

> Sometimes I don't follow the suggestions. For example, she says, 'You have to eat a certain amount of carbohydrates'. But sometimes, I don't want to eat pasta for lunch but I want to eat a salad, and I don't take insulin. I understand the advice of the doctor, but I don't always follow it. (DC-Pregnant, interview with a pregnant woman, 22 years old)

While self-tracking for remote management can be accepted and even appreciated, some minor deviations from the prescribed path show that what is at stake is not the mere data sharing but reaffirmation of an autonomous space for self-managing. This will be made more evident below.

Self-tracking for e-learning

Acquiring self-management skills is a continuous process that requires a significant effort by both patients and providers. Technologies and drugs change rapidly, and the time needed to educate patients is not compatible with the limited resources of the healthcare system. Adults with poorly controlled diabetes pose a significant challenge since they are supposed to be autonomous and sometimes decide not to go for routine examinations. One doctor noted that it was not uncommon to find that a patient was still using old devices or drugs or managing herself 'the old way', with poor results, despite all efforts. Also, children or their parents might suffer from insufficient education because doctors provided information only a little bit at a time on the assumption that delivering all of the needed information at once would be counterproductive.

The selection of children and adults with poorly controlled diabetes was intended to address this challenge. The clinicians considered the remote monitoring of self-tracked data as an opportunity to improve the self-care abilities of patients under the guidance of healthcare professionals and through the suggestions provided by the app.

> [Mother of Mario[2]]: Good morning, Doctor. We're struggling because Mario's blood sugar levels seem to follow their own logic absolutely independently from what we do. We've substituted 'rapid-acting insulin' with 'high rapid-acting insulin'. But Mario's blood sugar values increase during the night. Is it due to Mario's persistent cold?

> [Paediatric Doctor]: Dear [Mario's Mother], at around eleven in the evening, I'd keep [using] 'fast-acting insulin', increasing it by one unit. That's the sunset effect (increased insulin requirements from approximately six in the evening to two in the morning) typical of this age. Don't worry! (Paediatrics, messages between paediatrician and mother of a 7-year-old boy)

Parents of children who have had a recent diabetes onset are constantly faced with issues that they cannot address due to their limited experience. In the transition to autonomous management, they perceive themselves as being inexperienced and not yet able to manage their child's diabetes by themselves. Self-tracking and data sharing offer the opportunity to receive timely advice when parents have doubts about data interpretations and insulin therapy. Education may go hand in hand with a prescription, such as in the case in the above interview excerpt, where the change of therapy is used to illustrate a general rule. However, in self-tracking for e-learning, the emphasis is on providing information or 'tricks of the trade' that can be reused autonomously by patients.

> Hi Marco, do you know the 'rule of 15' to manage hypos? When you have a low glucose level, you need to eat 15 grams of sugar and then measure the glucose level again after 15 minutes, and if it's still under 100 [mg/dl], eat 15 grams more. If you are above 100 [mg/dl], you're fine. This will help with insulin peaks. P.S. Fifteen gr of sugar equal two sugar packets, three jellies, one fruit juice or half a can of Coke. (DC-Adults, message from nurse to patient)

This was a message frequently sent to adult patients by DC-Adults. As the trial progressed, it was discovered that most of the patients lacked the basic skills to treat recurring issues, and self-tracking allowed providers to pass on ready-to-use information. This discovery induced some clinicians to rethink the meaning of the system. While it had initially been considered a remote monitoring tool, some doctors and nurses came to see it as an instrument with which to assess the self-managing skills of patients and to deliver education in a timely and more effective fashion. However, this required asking patients to perform their self-tracking duties regularly, which proved to require a significant effort. Nurses spent some time every day not just on replying to messages or giving advice but also on reminding patients to input data or to acknowledge receiving the data. Although adult patients appreciated the education provided, they did not consider it necessary to maintain the relationship with the diabetes centre for the entire duration of the trial, and they decided to resume the usual self-management enriched by the experience acquired.

> [It's been useful] to know you're not alone. Now I don't feel alone even if I've stopped using the system. [This is] because the experience I've gained about food and knowledge about diabetes are good. I can manage myself. (DC-Adults, interview with a male patient, 24 years old)

It is not always easy for a patient to change his or her way of managing diabetes, especially if the patient has been autonomous for many years. In such cases, patients have developed solid knowledge, strategies and self-representations concerning illness management and, more generally, 'what is necessary in order to feel good'. Consequently, when adults with diabetes begin a new course of educational training, they may resist acquiring new forms of behaviour considered optimal in the medical community but perceived as intrusive by patients. In these processes, doctor–patient communication changes some self-management practices but seems not to affect others.

Self-tracking as boundary setting

During the disease's trajectory, diabetes management is marked by different phases characterised by different ways of relating with providers. After diabetes onset in children, there is a strong mandate for the doctor to educate the parents on the management of the disease. On the one hand, the healthcare professionals try to enhance the parents' self-management skills in order to reduce their workload; on the other, the parents often believe that 'good parents have to know how take care of their children'. Consequently, for parents who had developed basic self-management knowledge, the system was conceived as a support for self-care practices and, in particular, for care activities perceived as demanding (e.g. counting carbohydrates or calculating insulin bolus). Similarly, adults with 'bad' blood sugar values after a period of education by the hospital considered the system to be useful for improving their self-management skills. In these cases, self-tracking practices did not involve doctors: the patients recorded and interpreted clinical information autonomously. The choice to not share data asserted both the capacity for self-management and the capacity for interpretation and therapeutic action. Thus, the symbolic boundary between medical expertise and the experiential knowledge of patients and caregivers was reconstructed, thereby reaffirming the two different spheres of action.

> I personally wouldn't call the doctor [in the case of hypo- or hyperglycaemia] ... because I know why it has happened ... it's not carelessness, it's not negligence ... we consider ourselves quite conscientious ... we know how to evaluate things ... (Paediatrics, interview with the father of a 3-year-old diabetic child)

This boundary was defended with a refusal to synchronize data from the app to the server so that the patient could still see the data but was restricted from access to the department. During the trials, some patients used the system in a way that prevented doctors from intervening, and the technology became a way for the patients to reaffirm their autonomy in diabetes management. This was done by making selective use of the system: using the logbook and advanced functions but not answering doctors' messages. When doctors tried to intervene, they sometimes faced unpleasant reactions.

> I tried to send messages and, if they didn't answer, I phoned. But they were always 'sick' [blood sugar levels are higher for patients with influenza], and you come to realize that there's a wall. (Paediatrics, interview with a physician)

The metaphor of the 'wall' blocking communication expresses the unwillingness of some patients to redefine their relationship with the care provider. The patients who were 'behind the wall', so to speak, did not consider the use of messages to be useful; rather, they expressed their appreciation for those functions that could help their self-tracking become more effective and autonomous.

> I thought, 'Good!' I have a tool with which I can record blood sugar values and insulin doses and, moreover, I can see graphs of my trends. The strength of the system is its high customization. You can set the limits of hyper- and hypoglycaemia, the colours and the tables. (DC-Adults, interview with a male patient, 24 years old)

On the one hand, users in search of greater autonomy did not know the options designed for communication with doctors. On the other hand, when doctors tried to contact them, they used ploys to avoid the doctors' control or simply ignored messages left by the doctors.

Paradoxically, this use of the system was perfectly in line with the usual self-tracking and self-managing practices taught to these users since the very beginning of their healthcare trajectory. Once patients reached a significant degree of autonomy, they only had relationships with doctors in emergencies or during their periodic face-to-face visits, when they discussed the medium- and long-term consequences of their disease. The use of the system to increase one's own skills in self-management while restricting access to doctors was, thus, consistent with the reaffirmation of the boundaries.

Discussion

Drawing on the research described, we now focus on two main considerations: the selective use of self-tracking as a way to redefine a therapeutic alliance and the costs and meanings associated with 'pushed' self-tracking.

Redefining the therapeutic alliance through selective use of the system

We cannot ignore the facts that technologies are not neutral and that they do not come from nowhere. Designers inscribe programs of action in technical artefacts; but, as Latour notes (1992), artefacts in themselves cannot guarantee that the program will be carried out. Intended users of the system were not presented with a binary choice between use and non-use; rather, they could enact technology selectively to fit into their lives (Orlikowski, 2000).

Although the heads of the departments customised the system in order to establish stricter control and intervention, the emerging practices of use revealed that customisation was not enough to induce patients to engage in self-tracking as imagined by the providers. Some patients enacted the technology using only some selected functions. They did not synchronize data using the system as a self-tracking tool whose data were for personal use. While this may look like a resisting practice, it should be noted that the healthcare providers themselves were not always dissatisfied with the emerging practices. They redefined their expectations regarding the system by accepting that it was not to be seen as a monitoring tool but rather as an e-learning platform (DC-Adults) and as a support for autonomous management (Paediatrics).

Through the constant reproduction of patterns of use – a 'repetition without repetition' (Béguin & Clot, 2004) – while never discussing the system's meaning explicitly, patients and providers progressively defined a situated and contextual common understanding of the meaning of the technology and the self-tracking practices associated with its use (Gherardi, 2010; Suchman, Blomberg, Orr, & Trigg, 1999). Although self-tracking technologies can be designed with an agenda (Fox, 2015), their meaning cannot be determined *a priori*; rather, their connotation is the emerging and non-predictable outcome of the practices of which it becomes a part.

Pushing (clinical) self-tracking

Moving to the conclusions, some considerations follow with regard to the notion of 'pushed self-tracking', that is, self-tracking initiated in response to external encouragement (Lupton, 2014b). In this paper, we have focused on what we have called 'clinical self-tracking', which is a common practice in the shared management of chronic conditions like diabetes. The case analysed suggests that even if clinicians can 'push' self-tracking practices, they are not necessarily able to 'steer' them. While a distal view of pushing may represent it as a single activity (i.e. asking the patient to keep a logbook), on closer inspection, it seems more like a long-lasting process that requires time, patience and social skills. To keep the self-tracking practices going, care providers need to remind patients to input data and share them. They can strengthen the message either through positive reinforcement to a previous data input or through subtle threats. Despite all efforts, however, patients can refuse to comply, or they can self-track but not share the data, so that the care providers stop pushing.

Moreover, a request to self-track for the benefit of the care team can be perceived by patients as intrusive. In the case presented, patients had a long history of self-tracking, and they were required to share the information with the care providers. What the technology allowed, however, was access by the providers to data not just during the routine examinations but on a daily basis. In cases like diabetes, in which patients are educated to be the principal decision-makers (Funnell & Anderson, 2004), some patients may consider this access to be a breach of the therapeutic pact because they regard the data collected to be primarily for their own use and self-management (Piras & Zanutto, 2014).

Finally, pushing can endanger the long-standing relationships between patients and providers, which will continue after the trial. For both patients and providers, self-tracking is not a stand-alone practice; rather, it is part of a relationship that defines reciprocal duties, expectations and roles. Its meaning can be only understood as part of a larger set of arrangements. Both provider and patients act with the knowledge that their decisions about self-tracking (i.e. pushing it, refusing it) will affect their relationship as a whole.

Conclusions

When discussing healthcare technology, we are often confronted with two conflicting rhetorics of technological promises and their associated nightmares (Pols, 2012). Self-tracking technologies are no exception, being considered either the cornerstones of new forms of healthcare management (Rivera-Pelayo et al., 2012; Swan, 2012) or parts of an agenda of medicalisation of society to be resisted (Fox, 2015).

In this paper, we have tried to provide a less polarised and more nuanced representation of what is at stake by taking a grounded approach to health self-tracking. We focused our attention on what we called 'clinical self-tracking', a form of 'pushed self-tracking' (Lupton, 2014b) in which patient education is required, data are standardised, patients perform data analysis and tracking evolves over time. The new patient–provider relationship is the arrangement arising from an open-ended process that providers try to steer by customising the technologies and that patients contribute to through unexpected self-tracking practices. We identified three purposes of self-tracking: remote management, e-learning and boundary setting. The analysis reveals the fluid and contingent nature of these social practices and the difficulties of strictly classifying them. For instance, patients might start collecting data under pressure from doctors (pushed self-tracking) but refuse to share the data with providers (self-tracking as boundary setting), thus adopting a 'quantified-self-like' approach (private self-tracking).

This study reaffirms the benefits of empirically grounded theorising as a way to grasp the rich and evolving phenomenology of self-tracking practices. This approach would be particularly relevant for investigating self-tracking among those who might benefit most from digital health interventions (e.g. the elderly, low-income patients and patients excluded from healthcare) but are the least likely to make use of them.

Notes

1. Paediatrics: only one physician is in charge of all patients with diabetes. Unlike other departments involved in the trial, the physician does not work with a diabetes nurse, and he manages the system by himself. DC-Adult and DC-Pregnant: patients are assigned to a case manager (nurse) and one or two doctors.
2. Fictitious name.

Disclosure statement

No potential conflict of interest was reported by the authors.

Funding

This work was supported by Department of Health and Social Politics of the Autonomous Province of Trento (Italy) [TreC2 Project].

References

Allen, A. L. (2008). Dredging up the past: Lifelogging, memory, and surveillance. *The University of Chicago Law Review*, *75*(1), 47–74.

Ancker, J. S., Witteman, H. O., Hafeez, B., Provencher, T., Van de Graaf, M., & Wei, E. (2015). The invisible work of personal health information management among people with multiple chronic conditions: Qualitative interview study among patients and providers. *Journal of Medical Internet Research*, *17*(6), e137. http://www.jmir.org/2015/6/e137/

Bossewitch, J., & Sinnreich, A. (2013). The end of forgetting: Strategic agency beyond the panopticon. *New Media & Society*, *15*(2), 224–242.

Brennan, P. F., & Casper, G. (2015). Observing health in everyday living: ODLs and the care-between-the-care. *Personal and Ubiquitous Computing*, *19*(1), 3–8.

Béguin, P., & Clot, Y. (2004). L'action située dans le développement de l'activité. *Activités*, *1*(2), 35–50.

Conrad, P. (2007). *The medicalization of society*. Baltimore, MD: Johns Hopkins University Press.

Doyle, J., Walsh, L., Sassu, A., & McDonagh, T. (2014). Designing a wellness self-management tool for older adults: Results from a field trial of your wellness. In *Proceedings of the 8th international conference on pervasive computing technologies for healthcare*, edited by Andreas Hein, Susanne Boll, Friedrich Köhler (pp. 134–141). Brussels: Institute for Computer Sciences, Social-Informatics and Telecommunications Engineering.

Fox, N. J. (2015). Personal health technologies, micropolitics and resistance: A new materialist analysis. *Health: An Interdisciplinary Journal for the Social Study of Health, Illness and Medicine*.

Funnell, M. M., & Anderson, R. M. (2004). Empowerment and self-management of diabetes. *Clinical Diabetes*, *22*(3), 123–127.

Gherardi, S. (2010). Telemedicine: A practice-based approach to technology. *Human Relations*, *63*(4), 501–524.

King, N. (1998). Template analysis. In G. Symon & C. Cassel (Eds.), *Qualitative methods and analysis in organizational research: A practical guide* (pp. 118–134). Thousand Oaks, CA: Sage.

Latour, B. (1992). Where are the missing masses? The sociology of a few mundane artifacts. In W. Bijker & J. Law (Eds.), *Shaping technology-building society. Studies in sociotechnical change* (pp. 225–259). Cambridge: MIT Press.

Ledger, D., & McCaffrey, D. (2014). *Inside wearables: How the science of human behavior change offers the secret to long-term engagement.* Cambridge, MA: Endeavour Partners.

Li, I., Dey, A., & Forlizzi, J. (2010). *A stage-based model of personal informatics systems.* Proceedings of the SIGCHI Conference on Human Factors in Computing Systems, Atlanta.

Lupton, D. (2014a). Beyond techno-utopia: Critical approaches to digital health technologies. *Societies, 4*(4), 706–711.

Lupton, D. (2014b). *Self-tracking modes: Reflexive self-monitoring and data practices.* Available at SSRN: http://dx.doi.org/10.2139/ssrn.2483549

Lupton, D. (2016). Towards critical health studies: Reflections on two decades of research in Health and the way forward. *Health, 20*(1), 49–61.

MacLeod, H., Tang, A., & Carpendale, S. (2013). *Personal informatics in chronic illness management.* Paper presented at the Proceedings of Graphics Interface 2013.

Moen, A., & Brennan, P. F. (2005). Health@ Home: The work of health information management in the household (HIMH): Implications for consumer health informatics (CHI) innovations. *Journal of the American Medical Informatics Association, 12*(6), 648–656.

Orlikowski, W. J. (2000). Using technology and constituting structures: A practice lens for studying technology in organizations. *Organization Science, 11*(4), 404–428.

Oudshoorn, N. (2012). How places matter: Telecare technologies and the changing spatial dimensions of healthcare. *Social Studies of Science, 42*(1), 121–142.

Piras, E. M., & Zanutto, A. (2010). Prescriptions, X-rays and grocery lists. Designing a personal health record to support (the invisible work of) health information management in the household. *Computer Supported Cooperative Work (CSCW), 19*(6), 585–613.

Piras, E. M., & Zanutto, A. (2014). 'One day it will be you who tells us doctors what to do!'. Exploring the 'personal' of PHR in paediatric diabetes management. *Information Technology & People, 27*(4), 421–439.

Pols, J. (2012). *Care at a distance: On the closeness of technology.* Amsterdam: Amsterdam University Press.

Rivera-Pelayo, V., Zacharias, V., Müller, L., & Braun, S. (2012). Applying quantified self approaches to support reflective learning. In *Proceedings of the 2nd international conference on learning analytics and knowledge,* edited by Simon Buckingham Shum, Dragan Gasevic, Rebecca Ferguson (pp. 111–114). New York: ACM.

Suchman, L., Blomberg, J., Orr, J. E., & Trigg, R. (1999). Reconstructing technologies as social practice. *American Behavioral Scientist, 43*(3), 392–408.

Swan, M. (2012). Health 2050: The realization of personalized medicine through crowdsourcing, the quantified self, and the participatory biocitizen. *Journal of Personalized Medicine, 2*(3), 93–118.

Training to self-care: fitness tracking, biopedagogy and the healthy consumer

Aristea Fotopoulou and Kate O'Riordan

ABSTRACT
In this article, we provide an account of *Fitbit*, a wearable sensor device, using two complementary analytical approaches: auto-ethnography and media analysis. Drawing on the concept of biopedagogy, which describes the processes of learning and training bodies how to live, we focus on how users learn to self-care with wearable technologies through a series of micropractices that involve processes of mediation and the sharing of their own data via social networking. Our discussion is oriented towards four areas of analysis: data subjectivity and sociality; making meaning; time and productivity and brand identity. We articulate how these micropractices of knowing one's body regulate the contemporary 'fit' and healthy subject, and mediate expertise about health, behaviour and data subjectivity.

Introduction

In recent years, tracking devices and wearable sensors have come to occupy a key locus in the mediation of the healthy and responsible citizen. Application-based tracking services, such as *Map My Run,* and tracking sensors like *Fitbit* have become popular elements of consumer culture. Devices such as *Fitbit* are often framed in policy and in the media as enabling significant moves towards a healthy lifestyle, despite the fact that they are at the leisure end of a health-to-leisure spectrum of medical devices. They come together with the promotion of individual responsibility in health care policy (Beck & Beck-Gersheim, 2001) and 'healthy living' (Burrows, Nettleton, & Bunton, 1995). In this context, how is self-care being learned with the use of digital apps and wearable technologies? What kinds of subjectivities do self-tracking and data quantification enable? Drawing on the concept of biopedagogy, which describes the processes of learning and training bodies how to live, in this article, we examine *Fitbit*, a wearable sensor device, from two different analytical approaches: auto-ethnography and media analysis.

When it comes to *Fitbit* and other wearable devices there is more at stake than behavioural change and individual well-being. As we argue in this article, these are normative devices teaching users how to be good consumers and biocitizens. Users are offered training in self-care through wearable technologies through a series of micropractices that involve processes of mediation and sharing their own data via social networking.

Importantly, they learn to incorporate forms of ubiquitous computing and data literacy in their lives. This article focuses on how such new micropractices of self-caring and knowing oneself are disseminated through the media and the *Fitbit* platform itself. By employing the concept of digital biopedagogy, we articulate how these micropractices of knowing one's body through data regulate the contemporary fit and healthy subject.

Wearable devices are practiced as digital technologies of the body. They are also media texts, and therefore present an added layer of analytic complexity. It then becomes necessary to frame them both as artefacts with practices, and as communication devices that address users/audiences in particular ways. Hence our approach to *Fitbit* encompasses both the experiential dimensions of practising a wearable technology, and its symbolic and meaning-making dimensions as a digital communication device. This allows us to explore the idea of wearable technologies as pedagogic technologies that incorporate forms of training and knowledge production and which, in this process, create new meanings about the technology, as well as new expert/lay person identities. *Fitbit's* accumulation of personal data and use of social networking technologies indicate a shift of responsibility from the medical expert to the tracking technology and to the individual. Operating both through promotional media discourse about the device, and by the multiple address of the device as itself a discursive agent, this shift is often accentuated and articulated as a form of democratisation and individual empowerment.

Fitbit and biopedagogy

> My *Fitbit One* flashes that it will be out of battery soon and I am rushing to get to the charger and to a chair before it goes off. I'm worried that I will miss steps, that the graph will be incomplete, that there will be gaps. It seems that this tiny little piece of metal, gum and LCD screen has brought out an inner obsessiveness that I didn't know about, a compulsiveness to keep logs tidy and up-to-date. I genuinely crave for clean diagrams. (Field notes)

This auto-ethnographic field note introduces some our key questions: Why might people worry about their devices and have compulsive attachments to data visualisations that are continuous and do not contain information gaps? What else does using *Fitbit* teach people, and what have we learnt as researchers through different approaches?

Fitbit offers a range of wearable devices that can be attached to the wrist or clipped onto clothing. Daily use of *Fitbit* typically involves wearing the device throughout the day, while it monitors steps walked, floors climbed and calories burned. In some models (such as the model used in this study, Fitbit One) *Fitbit* offers additional features, such as sleep monitoring. The user needs to connect to the personal interface (referred to as the Dashboard) in order to upload the data logged by the device to the cloud-based system. This can happen through a website or mobile app; once logged in, the user can access charts with information of daily activity and compare their data over time or to other *Fitbit* users. Periodic synching is necessary for this update. In our study, the autoethnographer connected to the cloud at the end of every day. In addition to measuring data sensed directly by the device, by logging into the Dashboard the user can also enter details of food consumption and mood. The company suggests eating a specific amount of calories and walking a minimum of 10,000 steps a day in order to reach personal weight loss goals.

In what follows, we focus on the mode of address of digital health promotion and employ the concept of biopedagogy. Our interest is with the subjectivities that are being produced by the discourses that circulate in the media, and enabled through the design of the *Fitbit* interface of peripherals. Biopedagogy has been explored in health sociology to account for the ways in which truth and meaning about bodies are being constituted in multiple sites, such as policy documents, health promotion and the media (Wright & Harwood, 2009). Drawing from Foucault's classic work on biopower, and more recent work on pedagogy (see Bernstein, 2001; Bordo, 2003), Jan Wright and Valerie Harwood's edited volume on biopolitics and obesity focuses on the cultural beliefs, policies and other regulating and disciplinary practices that constitute pedagogies about how to live. Concentrating more on the media, Rail and Lafrance (2009) also use biopedagogy to analyse biopower when they account for the ways in which viewers of the reality television program *Nip and Tuck* are instructed how to think about the fat body. In these contexts, biopedagogy has been used primarily to think about how bodies are pathologised and disciplined and, more recently, how policy and market work in tandem to create the normative 'fit' and productive biocitizen (Rail & Jette, 2015). In this article, we are informed by these existing studies but we are also concerned with the biopedagogy of digital technologies and apps that operate in a pre-emptive mode. Like reality television and other cultural sites, *Fitbit* tracking devices mediate the body, prescribing what is normal and acceptable, including normal weight and weight loss through exercising and calorie restriction. The promotional media and the interface of the consumer device constitute biopedagogies about how to prevent the pathologised body and reproduce dominant discourses about the 'fit' and healthy body. Our attention is directed to the tensions between media representations, user experience, and knowledge-making about health promotion wearables, against the backdrop of economic cuts, austerity and the reshaping of the health sector throughout Europe. In this context, the rhetoric of crisis in the healthcare sectors, and fears that care may become unavailable to many, invite new modes of control over the body and health. Further, as we discuss in our analysis of the interface, *Fitbit* is designed to address users and consumers as learners of technology, instructed to incorporate self-logging in their everyday lives, making everyday practices productive. Thus, biopedagogy also relates to the new subjectivities that emerge in relation to what has been recently termed as 'datafication' (Mayer-Schönberger & Cukier, 2013) and 'dataveillance' (van Dijck, 2014).

Reviewing wearables: communication systems and social technologies

The emerging body of research around wearables has registered the centrality of locative devices, smart phone apps (Lupton, 2014b) and data repositories for healthcare (Gunnarsdottir et al., 2015; Mort, Roberts, & Callen, 2013; Oudshoorn, 2011). The quantified self (QS) is one example of a community of people who use wearable devices in order to log personal information and improve various aspects of personal life, such as mood, physical and mental performance, or other aspects of everyday life, such as air quality, and it has become a subject of critical thought (Bossewitch & Sinnreich, 2013, Fotopoulou, 2014; Shull, Jirattigalachote, Hunt, Cutkosky, & Delp, 2014). Insurance companies and employers routinely introduce wearables in the workplace as part of the well-being and health package deals they offer to their employees (Olson & Tilley, 2014). Although fitness and well-being wearables such as *Fitbit* are not intended as medical devices per se, they are part of an apparatus of digitised health promotion (Lupton, 2013, 2014a).

Digital health promotion strategies that largely emphasise individual responsibility disregard the social, cultural and political dimensions of digital technology use (Lupton, 2014a). We examine these social dimensions here, and indicate some of the implications of promoting self-reliance in relation to public health.

Wearable sensor technologies bring new challenges but also have continuity with older systems. They intersect with biometrics (measurements of the body), which could also include facial recognition, body temperature and perspiration levels. However, biometrics have been cast as dystopian surveillance technologies and received explicit criticism for the way in which they objectify bodies, with their limited set of biometric indexes (Magnet, 2011). Although these issues also apply to health promotion, here our focus is different. *Fitbit* wearables are central to what Deborah Lupton refers to as a 'data utopian discourse on the possibilities and potential of big data, metricisation and algorithmic calculation for healthcare' (2013, p. 14). Wearables are attached to imaginaries in which self-surveillance offers agency (Mann, 2005), and a utopian vision of a body that might escape pathology, if it is paired with technological expertise.

Methods

The media analysis included an analysis of the interface, and textual analysis of the promotional material. Initially, we undertook an exploratory textual analysis of news media of a total of 140 articles during a one-year period (April 2012–2013), which were clustered around health, leisure and lifestyle sections, as well as trade press.[1] We aimed to identify dominant, ambivalent and oppositional framings and meanings attributed to *Fitbit* through discourse analysis. We identified the language used to construct the device as meaningful, and the subject positions offered through these formulations. We derived the sample by searching for 'Fitbit', 'wearable', 'tracker' and 'sensor' as key terms through the Nexis news database. Of these articles only three significantly challenged the promotion of *Fitbit* as a 'cool' new device to help manage and control weight and wellness.

From the initial textual analysis it became evident that it was important to understand how the device can be used in everyday life, the subject positions that are enabled when bodies connect and interact with the technology, how the utopian/dystopian narratives in adopting wearable technologies map out during daily use, and how other key claims about expertise and knowledge are communicated through the interface design of the device. The textual analysis was thus complemented with an auto-ethnographic analysis and an interface analysis of *Fitbit*. The interface analysis involved examining the smartphone app, the device screen and the website, which are its key modes of communication and knowledge production.

For the small-scale auto-ethnographic methods, Fotopoulou used the *Fitbit* device and logged everyday physical activity, including sleep, for a period of three months. Auto-ethnography seeks to analyse personal experience as a source of knowledge and it privileges the self, situated in a particular cultural context, as a source of narrative (Bassett, 2012; Ellis, 2004; Ellis & Bochner, 2000). This was particularly relevant here since the use of self-logging technologies is about self-improvement. Daily use of the device included wearing it during the day and during sleep; trying to meet the manufacturer's generic suggestion to walk 10,000 steps per day; and logging into the personal interface (Dashboard) at the end of each day to check the data visualisations of the activity that had been logged. The autoethnographer joined a community of *Fitbit* users, which served as a common cultural identity. She kept reflexive ethnographic notes (quoted in this paper as field notes), which focused on how her understanding and approach to her own data and bodily functions changed with the use of *Fitbit*. These notes were developed further with the following key questions as guides: what kinds of knowledge are users invited to produce with the interface; how does the interpretative framework prescribed by the device allow users/consumers to make meaning about their own data, and what kinds of stories can they tell about themselves?

The combination of media analysis (interface analysis and textual analysis of news/promotional material) with auto-ethnography was important in order to approach the device and its operation as part of a wider promotion for digital health.

Analysis

Fitbit enables a range of meanings, literacies and forms of knowledge that are central to shaping certain subjectivities and consumer behaviours. Self-tracking with *Fitbit* involves a set of micropractices through which self-care is normalised as the way to be fit and healthy. These involve learning how to operate the device and how to make sense of the data, and they constitute a form of training.

'You can get this!' everyday coaching and making data social

In media coverage *Fitbit* appears overwhelmingly as an *app*. The terms 'gadget', 'device', 'gizmo' and 'wearable' are all used, but the term with the highest incidence is app. Much of the news coverage that we investigated deployed puns such as 'appy New Year'; 'appy days'; 'if you're appy and you know it', in the headlines. Through this language, an ecology of mobiles, smart phones and wearables is evoked. This framing helps to locate the *Fitbit* as a dimension of digital culture and to emphasise it as a networked object.

In use, the screen of the device worn on the body displays numerical information about fitness activity, such as steps walked, floors climbed and calories burnt. In addition to this information, the screen periodically displays messages that aim to create a sense of connection with the user, and at the same time, establish the device in its role as a sports-trainer (for instance 'love ya Mary' or 'you can get this!'). This display of motivational messages on the device screen and on the interface dashboard introduces a form of coaching, which is ongoing even when the device is not actually connected to the wireless interface.

The offline sociality of motivational messages is complemented with what has become standard online connectivity: the app and website are similar to others (activity tracking, calorie measuring) in their use of social networking functions, such as profile, friends and groups (see boyd & Ellison, 2007 for a thorough analysis of these functions). These social networking functions, and the basic communication on the screen of the device, are integral aspects of how knowledge about the body and the technology is acquired and exchanged through the *Fitbit* interface, and a key way in which health is digitally mediated.

Since self-measurement is the focus of the *Fitbit* interface, it could be said that sociality and connectivity are not directly necessary. Therefore the design features that enable sociality and connectivity in the interface could be considered as a marketing strategy that renders *Fitbit* 'as if' social: the social networking elements are used to render the interface attractive to users, when the primary aim, as with other similar health-related businesses and cloud-based tracking devices, is the collection of personal data from the user (see Atzori, Carboni, & Iera, 2014). Indeed, *Fitbit* prompts users to consent to share their recorded data with the Microsoft Health Vault (https://www.healthvault.com/gb/en), which is a central node for sharing health information on Windows 8. Currently *Fitbit* provides interested users with an application program interface should they wish to download their raw data but premium membership is required. However, making the data meaningful in another context requires good technical knowledge. Thus *Fitbit* offers a data subjectivity that is 'social' but limited. It mainly teaches people how to be subject to data, or data participants, while it offers a possibility of empowered data subjectivity.

Self-tracking is fun: numbers and metaphors

The user is presented with information about their fitness in two ways: through an interpretation of the quantified data input and manual data entry in the form of infographics and text (see Figure 1); and through the game features, which come in the form of badges and levels. For example, the *Fitbit One* depicts a flower that grows bigger the more active you are (Figure 2).

The analysis of the data is statistical and cumulative. Bodily information about weight, age and height is provided by the user and can be shared with other users with the 'friends' function. The range of information that can be shared with friends in *Fitbit* is determined by the platform (food, activities, weight, sleep, mood and allergies). A 'Journal' feature allows for diary-type prose content to be recorded and shared. The diagrams display the average score since the beginning of the use, as well as peaks and lows of an activity during the same day. However, these infographics cannot be further manipulated or read in much detail. *Fitbit* allows for an accessible and limited mode of knowledge acquisition and subjectivity, which is playful and 'fun'.

Quantified accounts are expressed through numbers, which are made meaningful through contextualisation and interpretation. *Fitbit* offers a strong interpretative framework and visual interface with the online account. This way it creates a set of visual cues and narrative elements for the user to interpret these numbers. It compares user

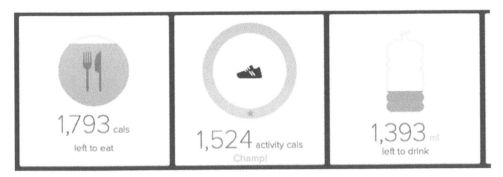

Figure 1. *Fitbit* dashboard showing tiles for food, steps and water: part of the app interface.

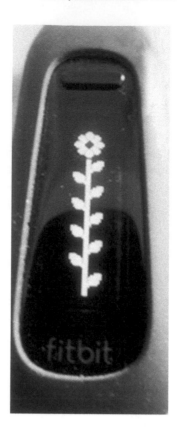

Figure 2. Fitbit One's flower.

measurements to certain targets, either set through *Fitbit's* health promotion formula (10,000 steps daily, two litres of water) or by the user as goals. These are illustrated through real or fictional images. For example, during the auto-ethnography, climbing an estimated height of 16 building floors was represented as climbing the height of God-zilla. With a film reference and a comparison to a fictional creature, *Fitbit* aims to enhance the experience of self-tracking by providing an additional path to self-understanding and pleasure from the user's engagement with data. The key framing here is that learning to self-track is fun and that fun is a new way of dealing with the 'serious' world of health.

Fitbit further cultivates sociality and competitive play with the use of badges and levels. These operate as motivational tools and are a recognisable marketing strategy, in which game elements (e.g. reward structures, positive reinforcement and challenges) are inte-grated in non-gaming contexts (see Zichermann & Cunningham, 2011 for more about 'gamification' as marketing strategy). There is a new generation of immersive running games that aims to motivate behavioural change in users. Game design in healthcare in particular aims to encourage users towards a model of self-management (see Swan, 2009). This element of gamification of everyday practices that characterises *Fitbit* is common in self-quantification (Till, 2014).

The sociality and motivational cues offered by *Fitbit* are only generated by compliance. While learning about oneself appears to be social, a form of camaraderie, in fact it intro-duces what Rail and Jette have called 'neo-authoritarianism' (2015, p. 328) in the shape of a digital coach. There are no badges or motivational prompts for inactivity or missed data, but there are red warning zones in the infographics for failing to meet consumption and activity targets. Although, in other platforms, users rely on paid subscriptions for punishment if they do not train enough or overeat (Cederström & Spicer, 2015), in *Fitbit* the emphasis is not on punitive language or warnings; it is on reward, and motivation. The use of fun and play, and the emphasis on positivity is also a way of navigating the threat of an implicit dystopian imaginary in which health care is unavailable. The connected, continuous collection of data from sensors and the sharing of these data in social networks are instrumental for the operationalisation of this model, and interface design is key for adoption in everyday life.

'A gap in my graph!' temporality and learning to be productive

Fitbit generates data through a selection of specific points so a judgement about what counts as productive biological information is built into the design of the device. *The Sun's* (highly popular UK redtop newspaper) assessment was that of 'a slimming aid' explaining that 'it counts the number of steps you take each day and converts the data into calories burnt'. This way of characterising biological data – as generated by counting walking, running, biking and swimming activities – together with calorie intake and weight measurements is the feature of *Fitbit* that is most dominant in media coverage. It is represented as a device that will manage body weight and active lifestyle through the mechanism of measurement, saving time by collecting data. A trend in the January 2013 coverage, picking up on press releases, was to link the device to getting more active after Christmas. Some articles picked up on the promise that *Fitbit* also offers a route into a health revolution, or links to a quantified self-movement, by referencing the capacity to put the *Fitbit* together with other databases. However, these references were rare and although *Fitbit* was used to anchor a prospective vision it stood in as sign for this future vision rather than providing evidence for such a system.

> Wearing the Fitbit has made me aware of my day and night cycles and temporal rhythms in a different way. Although monitoring bodily activity remained in the domain of the technology, I had an extra responsibility of wearing the *Fitbit* device at all times. My perception of time changed. It became the time of the diagram, the time of continuity and bundles of activity. When I failed to transfer the device from one pair of trousers to another, and in the meantime I climbed stairs a couple of times, this continuity was spoilt, there was a gap in my graph, like a gap in my performance. (Field notes)

These gaps in performance during Fotopoulou's experience of using *Fitbit One* registered as anxiety accompanied with thoughts such as 'what was I doing during this time?' In 'Pressed for time', Wajcman (2014) suggests that the acceleration of technological innovation in digital capitalism has made us feel that we are short of time in the increasingly busy lives we are leading. Multitasking, she explains, with digital devices has made leisure time disappear. Indeed with *Fitbit*, becoming and staying fit and healthy is a task that occurs around the clock because the collection of data takes place during work, leisure and sleep. No time is wasted; all time is productive, as long as you are alive to generate biological signals. From Fotopoulou's experience of using Fitbit, she observed that although *Fitbit* could have been useful in the long term with being mindful about the body, during the three months of use things just felt *busier*, as if there was always a task at hand. Arguably, doing auto-ethnography for a research project expanded working hours and acknowledging this context of monitoring is important:

> Would I have felt that I was excelling in working performance even when I used *Fitbit* after the time period of data collection for the research project? I continued using *Fitbit* after the autoethnographic period ended. Self-tracking *correctly* (without data gaps) felt good – I felt a sense of accomplishment. (Field notes)

A desire to be a 'good' monitoring subject (which in practice meant recording movement, climbing steps and keeping mobile during the day) was not only triggered by loyalty as a working researcher; as Wajcman (2014) notes, being busy, harried and short for time is a form of status amongst middle class professionals in contemporary digital capitalism. Being busy with self-quantifying and staying fit is a reassuring and rewarding form of capital, which might explain why people happily and voluntarily chose to labour and be productive as a lifestyle, outside working hours (cf. Gregg, 2011). Quantification is also a form of mediation between individual workers who do not connect in other ways in conditions of neoliberal precarity (Moore & Robinson, 2015). Thus being a productive subject with *Fitbit* concerns both the production of one's own health, through an imagination of being proactive and also the production of meaningful data. Continuous productivity is a key element of data subjectivity.

'The future is here': learning about the brand

In addition to self-knowledge about fitness activity, *Fitbit* encourages users to become more knowledgable about the *Fitbit* technology and brand, and therefore contribute to building a strong consumer/business relationship. The Community panel, perhaps the most social of all *Fitbit* elements, supports participation in discussion threads that relate almost exclusively to the use of the device, health, diet and medical discourses. So as pedagogic technologies, fitness wearables affirm self-logging and behavioural change, whilst facilitating belonging in both fitness and techno-savvy networked knowledge communities.

In UK print news, coverage occurred primarily in feature and review sections, and largely consisted of reproductions of press releases from consumer electronic shows and from *Fitbit* and its distributers' promotional material. Thus, most material was positive in some way. In much of this coverage, big visions were laid out so that *Fitbit* often operated to anchor much grander visions of innovation and futures. Headlines and framings included: 'Wearable revolution' 'revolutionising healthcare' 'electronic health record revolution' 'the future is here'. These stories ranged through a spectrum of prospective visions about medicine, or the consumer electronics market transformed, while referencing *Fitbit* as an example.

The *Fitbit* brand identity then is, on the one hand, a fun, cool gadget and, on the other hand, part of a vision of electronic health records, telemedicine and big data. The following quote from a trade press article in which *Fitbit* is promoted as 'pre-wired for the electronic health record revolution' is from *Medical Marketing and Media* under the headline 'Devices and Diagnostics: The App Avant-Garde':

> one of the advance guard of a new breed of medical device-one that's part app and part gizmo and interfaces with smartphones to allow patients with chronic conditions like diabetes an

easy, DIY way of monitoring their health and sharing that data with their doctors. It's a tool tailor-made for this era of Big Data, empowered patients and ever fewer primary care physicians, who have less time. (Arnold, 2012, n.p.)

This broad vision of 'empowered patients' comes from the USA, but is also taken up in the UK and European contexts, where a vision of empowered patients comes together with cuts in public health care resources. Health and medical sectors are looking to digital media to decentralise and individualise the costs of health care. This reformulation of the citizen/consumer as a prospective informed patient operating in a hopeful economy of biological citizenship has been well documented in the sociology of health and medicine (Rabinow, 1996; Rose & Novas, 2005). The critical literature on obesity, particularly Wright and Harwood (2009), examines how this dovetails with the reduction in public health care budgets.

The *Fitbit* vision is thus part of two broader intersecting discourses. First, the self is made up in part through personal engagement with knowledge about biology. In this discourse of biological citizenship, a key issue the type of most relevant biological knowledge to assist in a project of self-making. What data should be collected and how can it be interpreted? *Fitbit* and other tracking devices compete for intelligibility of data and interpretation, and embody decisions about what biological data points are relevant. In this sense, they already offer forms of interpretation and meaning-making, like more traditional media texts. The second discourse is the one in which self-health care is increasingly important, as public front line resources dwindle. Here questions of cost, relevance, robustness of information and ease of use are important. In this paradigm, self-tracking offers a sort of technological fix to austerity.

Although there were many references to the mundane, even annoying rituals of data collection, criticisms of *Fitbit* only appeared in a minority (2%) of the news coverage analysed. These positioned self-monitoring as a kind of labour; data generation as pollution; privacy an area of concern and suggested that just measuring might not amount to managing health. Thus, a small fraction of the coverage challenged the frames provided in the *Fitbit* and consumer electronics promotional material and went further than merely trivialising the device. The most critical assessment of *Fitbit* positioned the device as part of broader data industry with the following headline: 'Your body isn't a temple, it's a data factory emitting digital exhaust' (Mardawi, 2013). This article drew on similar sources to the more positive review articles, namely press releases from consumer electronic shows about a future of biosenors linked to data infrastructure, but coupled these with reports that the French government was proposing a data tax that could be applied to companies profiting from user generated data.

Fitbit data: biopedagogy, self-tracking and datafied self

What is learnt from *Fitbit* data? Reading the data back to oneself, provides an account of how to move, how much to sleep and eat. In other words the collection of fitness data is a micropractice with a pedagogical dimension that concerns normalising and disciplining bodies. This biopedagogy is not simply about being 'fit' and well; it influence beliefs, behaviours and policies. It produces reality, as Foucault puts it when he explains biopower; 'it produces domains of objects and rituals of truth' (1991, p. 194). The pedagogic aspect of governmentality in fitness data tracking concerns a process of learning the behaviours and dispositions of self-care that are within acceptable modes of conduct in a neoliberal health landscape. The quote 'taking care of oneself requires knowing ... oneself' (Foucault, 1997, p. 283) presupposes a didactic process.

Beck and Beck-Gersheim (2001) have noted how in the age of genetics, being and staying healthy is framed as desirable and expected, beyond previous limits. It is indeed a 'voluntary compulsion' (144), based on the normative premise that more information will allow individuals to take better decisions for their health and that of their children. As is evidenced in the analysis above, *Fitbit* data contribute to the normalisation of self-monitoring and self-improvement, not only by establishing a firm regime of self-monitoring but also by offering new public sites where these practices are being sanctioned and affirmed (social media). The types of information made available to the *Fitbit* user can be thought of as encouraging an emerging self-management scheme and behaviour whereby users measure their bodily activity for productivity, learn from their own data and adjust their way of life accordingly.

Although logging information and checking stats is a mundane and often tedious activity (see user reviews, e.g. Waltz, 2012), it is at the same time a form of ritual (Couldry, 2003) involving positive affirmation. Through this, users re-assure themselves that they are being proactive and taking responsibility for their own well-being, in other words meeting the vision of the 'empowered patient' which, as noted above, is largely communicated in the media. The free labour demanded of the user who is self-tracking in order to sustain something that appears relatively simple and unmediated involves multiple modes of engagement, such as reading (interpreting) and sharing their own data via social networking. We can think of this as a wider symptom of the mediated contexts of life today, where services such as the collection of statistical data and health information are increasingly produced at home and given by users for free (see also Beer & Burrows, 2007). While there is ambivalence as to how far the collection of big data is an exploitative process (see for instance Couldry, Fotopoulou, & Dickens, 2016; Ritzer & Jurgenson, 2010; Tapscott & Williams, 2008), or a development to be celebrated, as is the case with the QS (Nafus & Sherman, 2014), this phenomenon has important ethical, political and social implications.

Learning self-responsibility and becoming an expert in self-care

Fitbit (and its fun-focused interface for the logging and accessing of personal data) seems to fit in a social and political context of self-responsibility. State approaches to health in the age of austerity that link to conservative policies throughout Europe and America can be considered within a wider context and historical stronghold of neoliberalism as an ideology. In the UK, where there is generalised access to the welfare system, responsibilising the self has been a key governance strategy characterising neoliberal policy since Margaret Thatcher's administration in the 1980s. Entrenched by New Labour's Third Way politics in the 1990s, it emphasised flexible employment and life-long learning (Besley & Peters, 2007). This has meant intensification of moral regulation, privatisation and limiting the State's role in favour of responsibilising the individual to invest in their own education and welfare: both an economic and moral process (Peters, 2001). More recently, as De Vogli (2011) notes, neoliberal policy responses to the economic crisis by national governments and the G-20, targeting the health sector specifically, have resulted in increasing mortality, health and economic inequalities between and within countries.

The result of such policies is a shift of emphasis from medical professionals services to self-empowerment. Health moves from the visible economy of the medical industries and the state to the less visible sphere of consumer labour. In the community sections of *Fitbit*, users predominately discuss medical issues and link to further sources of knowledge. This mode of engagement encourages users to participate and share, and to interact with other *Fitbit* users for information and personal development. Instead of relying on a physician or other professionals, the user is offered a mode of self-reliance coupled with support from the *Fitbit* user community. Thus, the encouragement of a consumer-knowledge community operates within a larger assumption and normalisation of digital connectivity and social networking. Digital health promotion and biopedagogy work together, both by addressing users and consumers as learners of technology for self-care, and by instructing them that such technologies and digital online practices may offer a form of expertise.

Expertise here refers to becoming expert in one's use of wearables and one's own capacity to care for one's own well-being: becoming 'expert' in self-care with the use of wearable technologies. This can be thought to actively lend to what has been termed as 'e-scaped medicine' by Nettleton and Burrows (2003), a new medical cosmology whereby information and communication technologies are central as means of acquiring knowledge. Nettleton and Burrows (2003) view the internet as the social technology that assists with the task of reflexive management of risk, at a time of waning faith in medical 'experts'. In this view, the digitisation of the welfare state and e-health services is an advancement based on the assumption that more access to information is better for citizens, patients and consumers.

With *Fitbit*, and more generally within the new cultural context of self-tracking, the sheer volume of information is specifically about one's own activity and engagement with the technology. Instead of thinking about expertise and agency in relation to the proliferation of abstract knowledge sources online, here we observe the encouragement of focusing on one's own bodily production and online community (linked to the commercial device) as the source of such information and expertise. The QS motto 'self-knowledge through numbers' refers to such knowledge, founded on intentional accumulation of statistical data, rather than general health information about conditions and symptoms.

Conclusion

In this article, the framework of biopedagogy provides a way of analysing a series of micro-practices that mediate expertise about health and shape data subjectivity. The pedagogic aspect of governmentality in self-tracking assumes learning the behaviours and dispositions of self-care, which constitute acceptable modes of conduct in a neoliberal health landscape. Our discussion focuses on four areas of analysis: data subjectivity and sociality; time and productivity; making meaning around data and brand identity.

With *Fitbit*, data are made social. Data subjectivity is 'fun' but limited, and it requires being always productive, even during sleep. Thinking about productivity in relation to temporality in particular links to a broader discourse of the ideal proactive consumer of self-tracking health technologies. This proactive consumer and data subject makes meaning with numbers in the context of digital coaching, gamification and metaphor, as they feature in the *Fitbit* interface. Through the marketing interfaces of the *Fitbit* device, including reviews and device screens, consumers are invited to participate in a form of training, not only in the collection of data, and health awareness, but also in the technology itself. The ideal consumer and biocitizen of the digitised welfare state is expert in their own body data production, which provides them with a sense of agency about their health.

Data collection devices sell by presenting 'data collection as an always already good and productive practice' (Gardner & Wray, 2013, p. np). Trust in the objectivity of data and quantified methods, or dataism as van Dijck (2014) calls it, solidifies new modes of expertise. We may consequently think of a diffraction of expertise: from platforms (that set the protocols of health), through to bodies (that generate data in compliance with these protocols), back through the platforms (that provide the interpretation of the data); a recursive loop that opens up more markets for devices that track data. The fact that *Fitbit* wearables, and other commercial tracking devices, are promoted as leisure and fitness devices places them in the category of knowledge-for-prevention, which is also experiential and personal. An important question that arises then is how these experiential and embodied knowledges might resist the biopower of data.

Note

1. This article does not provide a substantive gender analysis. However, our news coverage analysis showed that *Fitbit* is targeted through health and lifestyle marketing towards young women as a lifestyle accessory. The full range of devices that record and measure activity and health-related data points are gendered in similar ways to the broader lifestyle market. That is to say that both men and women are targeted but women are targeted more heavily, and through different devices. For example, the *Fitbit One* shows a flower and the *Fitbit Flex* is smaller and more colourful and signified as 'flex' – elements usually positioned on women in promotional materials. The *Fitbit Charge* is chunkier, black or grey and signified as 'charge' and is usually positioned on men with some shots of women.

Disclosure statement

No potential conflict of interest was reported by the authors.

Funding information

The research leading to this publication has received funding from the European Community's Seventh Framework Programme (FP7/2007–2013) [grant agreement number 288971] EPINET. Coordinated by the Centre for the Study of the Sciences and Humanities, Allegt. 34 7800 Bergen Norway.

References

Arnold, M. (2012, June 1). *Devices and diagnostics: The App Avant-Garde.* Medical marketing and media. Retrieved from http://www.mmm-online.com/features/devices-diagnostics-the-app-avant-garde/article/241992/

Atzori, L., Carboni, D., & Iera, A. (2014). Smart things in the social loop: Paradigms, technologies, and potentials. *Ad Hoc Networks, 18,* 121–132.

Bassett, C. (2012). The real estate of the trained-up self: (Or is this *England*?). In R. Wilken & G. Goggin (Eds.), *Mobile technology and place* (pp. 104–122). New York, NY: Routledge.

Beck, U., & Beck-Gersheim, E. (2001). *Individualization: Institutionalized individualism and its social and political consequences.* London: Sage.

Beer, D., & Burrows, R. (2007). Sociology and, of and in Web 2.0: Some initial considerations. *Sociological Research Online, 12*(5), 17.

Bernstein, B. (2001). From pedagogies to knowledges. In A. Morais, I. Neves, B. Davies, & H. Daniels (Eds.), *Towards a sociology of pedagogy. The contribution of basil Bernstein to research* (pp. 363–368). New York, NY: Peter Lang.

Besley, T., & Peters, M. A. (2007). *Subjectivity & truth: Foucault, education, and the culture of self* (Vol. 303). New York: Peter Lang.

Bordo, S. (2003). *Unbearable weight: Feminism, western culture and the body* (10th ed.). Berkeley: University of California Press.

Bossewitch, J., & Sinnreich, A. (2013). The end of forgetting: Strategic agency beyond the panopticon. *New Media and Society, 15*(2), 224–242.

boyd, d., & Ellison, N. B. (2007). Social network sites: Definition, history, and scholarship. *Journal of Computer-Mediated Communication, 13*(1), 210–230.

Burrows, R., Nettleton, S., & Bunton, R. (1995). Sociology and health promotion. Health, risk and consumption under late modernism. *The Sociology of Health Promotion, 1*, 1–12.

Cederström, C., & Spicer, A. (2015). *The wellness syndrome.* London: John Wiley & Sons.

Couldry, N. (2003). *Media rituals: A critical approach.* London: Routledge.

Couldry, N., Fotopoulou, A., & Dickens, L. (2016). Real social analytics: A contribution towards a phenomenology of a digital world. *The British Journal of Sociology.* doi:10.1111/1468-4446.12183

De Vogli, R. (2011). Neoliberal globalisation and health in a time of economic crisis. *Social Theory and Health, 9*, 311–325.

van Dijck, J. (2014). Datafication, dataism and dataveillance: Big data between scientific paradigm and ideology. *Surveillance and Society, 12*(2), 197–208.

Ellis, C. (2004). *The ethnographic I: A methodological novel about autoethnography.* Walnut Creek, CA: AltaMira Press.

Ellis, C., & Bochner, A. P. (2000). Autoethnography, personal narrative, reflexivity. In Norman K. Denzin & Yvonna S. Lincoln (Eds.), *Handbook of qualitative research* (2nd ed., pp. 733–768). Thousand Oaks, CA: Sage. *Fitbit.* Retrieved from http://www.fitbit.com/uk/home

Foucault, M. (1991). *Discipline and punish: The birth of a prison.* London: Penguin.

Foucault, M. (1997). *Essential works of Foucault, Vol. 1: Ethics, subjectivity and truth.* New York: New Your Press.

Fotopoulou, A. (2014). *The quantified self community, lifelogging and the making of 'smart' publics.* Open Democrarcy. Participation Now, September 10. Retrieved February 22, 2015, from http://www.opendemocracy.net/participation-now/aristea-fotopoulou/quantified-self-community-lifelogging-and-making-of-'smart'-pub

Gardner, P., & Wray, B. (2013). From lab to living room: Transhumanist imaginaries of consumer brain wave monitors. *Ada: A Journal of Gender, New Media and Technology, 3.* n.p.

Gregg, M. (2011). *Work's intimacy.* Cambridge: Polity press.

Gunnarsdottir, K., Dijk, N., Fotopoulou, A., Guimarães Pereira, Â, O'Riordan, K., Rommetveit, K., & Vesnic-Alujevic, L. (2015). *Gadgets on the move and in stasis: Consumer and medical electronics, what's the difference? (Summary of findings and policy recommendations).* Lancaster: Lancaster University.

Lupton, D. (2013). The digitally engaged patient: Self-monitoring and self-care in the digital health era. *Social Theory and Health, 11*, 256–270.

Lupton, D. (2014a). Health promotion in the digital era: A critical commentary. *Health Promotion International, 30*(1), 174–183. doi:10.1093/heapro/dau091

Lupton, D. (2014b). Apps as artefacts: Towards a critical perspective on mobile health and medical apps. *Societies, 4*, 606–622.

Magnet, S. (2011). *When biometrics fail: Gender, race, and the technology of identity.* Durham, NC: Duke University Press.

Mann, S. (2005). Sousveillance and cyborglogs: A 30-year empirical voyage through ethical, legal, and policy issues. *Presence: Teleoperators and Virtual Environments, 14*(6), 625–646.

Mardawi, A. (2013). Your body isn't a temple, it's a data factory emitting digital exhaust. *The Guardian*, p. 25.

Mayer-Schönberger, V., & Cukier, K. (2013). *Big data: A revolution that will transform how we live, work, and think*. London: John Murray.

Moore, P., & Robinson, A. (2015). The quantified self: What counts in the neoliberal workplace. *New Media and Society*. doi:10.1177/1461444815604328

Mort, M., Roberts, C., & Callen, B. (2013). Ageing with telecare: Care or coercion in austerity? *Sociology of Health and Illness*, *35*(6), 799–812.

Nafus, D., & Sherman, J. (2014). This one does not go up to eleven: The quantified self movement as an alternative big data practice. *International Journal of Communication*, *8*, 1784–1794.

Nettleton, S., & Burrows, R. (2003). E-scaped medicine? Information, reflexivity and health. *Critical Social Policy*, *23*(2), 165–185.

Olson, P., & Tilley, A. (2014, April 17). The quantified other: Nest and Fitbit chase a lucrative side business. *Forbes*. Retrieved from http://www.forbes.com/sites/parmyolson/2014/04/17/the-quantified-other-nest-and-Fitbit-chase-a-lucrative-sidebusiness/

Oudshoorn, N. (2011). *Telecare technologies and the transformation of healthcare*. Houndmills: Palgrave Macmillan.

Peters, M. A. (2001). *Poststructuralism, marxism, and neoliberalism: Between theory and politics*. Lanham: Rowman & Littlefield.

Rabinow, P. (1996). *Essays on the anthropology of reason*. Princeton: Princeton University Press.

Rail, G., & Jette, S. (2015). Reflections on biopedagogies and/of public health: On Bio-others, rescue missions, and social justice. *Cultural Studies ↔ Critical Methodologies*, *15*(5), 327–336.

Rail, G., & Lafrance, M. (2009). Confessions of the flesh and biopedagogies: Discursive constructions of obesity on nip/tuck. *Medical Humanities*, *35*, 76–79.

Ritzer, G., & Jurgenson, N. (2010). Production, consumption, prosumption: The nature of capitalism in the age of the digital 'prosumer'. *Journal of Consumer Culture*, *10*(1), 13–36.

Rose, N., & Novas, C. (2005). Biological citizenship. In A. Ong & S. Collier (Eds.), *Global assemblages: Technology, politics and ethics as anthropological problems* (pp. 439–463). Malden, MA: Blackwell.

Shull, P.B., Jirattigalachote, W., Hunt, M.A., Cutkosky, M.R., & Delp, S. (2014). Quantified self and human movement: A review on the clinical impact of wearable sensing and feedback for gait analysis and intervention. *Gait and Posture*, *40*(1), 11–19. doi:10.1016/j.gaitpost.2014.03.189

Swan, M. (2009). Emerging patient-driven health care models: An examination of health social networks, consumer personalized medicine and quantified self-tracking. *International Journal of Environmental Research and Public Health*, *6*(2), 492–525.

Tapscott, D., & Williams, A. D. (2008). *Wikinomics: How mass collaboration changes everything*. London: Portfolio.

Till, C. (2014). Exercise as labour: Quantified self and the transformation of exercise into labour. *Societies*, *4*(3), 446–462.

Wajcman, J. (2014). *Pressed for time: The acceleration of life in digital capitalism*. Chicago: University of Chicago Press.

Waltz, E. (2012, September). *How I quantified myself: Can self measurement gadgets help us live better and healthier lives*. IEEE Spectrum. Retrieved from http://spectrum.ieee.org/biomedical/devices/how-i-quantified-myself

Wright, J., & Harwood, V. (2009). *Biopolitics and the 'obesity epidemic': Governing bodies*. New York: Routledge.

Zichermann, G., & Cunningham, C. (2011). *Gamification by design: Implementing game mechanics in web and mobile apps*. Sebastopol, CA: O'Reilly Media.

Harm reduction and the ethics of drug use: contemporary techniques of self-governance

Margaret Pereira and John Scott

ABSTRACT

Drawing on Foucault's conceptualisation of power, this paper examines public health as a distinctly modern regime of governance. An account of the historical regulation of drug use is traced in order to examine socio-historical shifts and lines of continuity in contemporary technologies of harm reduction. Using qualitative interview data, we examined practices of power in the context of contemporary drug use, including self-governance using techniques of monitoring, self-management and self-tracking. Participants' accounts revealed that they were encouraged to self-govern their drug use through a variety of reformist technologies that are embedded in harm-reduction programs. It is argued that participants' subjectivity is formed at the intersection of authoritative governance and self-governance, through ethical practices of the self which have emerged from disciplinary health practices, and incorporate the body as the site of power. We illustrate this by drawing a distinction between *hygienist* and *sanitationist* practices of public health. These governmental practices, which are embedded in public health programs, encourage people who use drugs to transform themselves into moral citizens, aligning their ethical practices with governing interests.

Introduction

This paper builds on existing post-structuralist accounts of health regulation by examining the development and operation of public health as a historically specific apparatus of power. Specifically, we seek to locate self-tracking within contemporary regimes of public health as techniques of self-governance. We examine public health as a regime of power that primarily invests in the body and operates from within the body. Lupton (2013, 2014) notes that self-tracking involves varied practices, some of which we argue here may be articulated with sovereign and disciplinary forms of power.

Much of the literature on self-tracking has emphasised digital technologies, which, with the advent of Web 2.0, have articulated what has been referred to as a quantified self (Lupton, 2015; Patron, Hansen, Fernandez-Luque, & Lau, 2012; Swan, 2012, 2013). While technology has assisted in the dispersal of self-tracking practices to broad populations, such practices trace their roots to a modern desire for 'good' health that is at once self-predicated and a social objective. While contemporary self-tracking practices often involve digital technologies, and detailed measurement and sharing of data, self-tracking has been closely aligned with biopolitical governance (Lupton, 2014) and, therefore, can be situated within the broader history of biopolitical technologies. We challenge socio-historical accounts of health regulation that assume that particular forms of domination become redundant at specific historical junctures. In doing so, we emphasise lines of continuity between historical shifts in the practice of power and the contemporary governance of drug use. With reference to drug use, we examine how current regimes of public health deploy technologies which utilise *both* practices of the self and practices of domination, taking the ethical self and social body as their site of governance. This is highlighted by drawing a distinction between what we term *sanitationist* and *hygienist* practices of public health.

Drawing on interview data from people who use drugs, we examine contemporary aspects of public health with reference to the management of drug use. In doing so we provide insights into how the governance of illicit drugs intersects with self-governance, using ethical techniques of self-monitoring, self-management, surveillance and self-tracking. In contemporary regimes of public health, people who use drugs are encouraged to engage in harm-reduction practices in order to improve health and achieve social and economic participation. Following post-structuralist accounts of the 'new public health', this paper locates these contemporary self-governance technologies within broader objectives of self-optimisation, using disciplinary health practices which constitute the body as the object and subject of power.

Theorising power and public health

Post-structuralist accounts of health regulation have been critical of attempts to make totalising or essentialist claims about the operation of power, and have instead examined *how* multiple localities and institutions of power have been instrumental in the production and governance of the 'healthy' body (see Adkins, 2001; Nettleton, 1997; Petersen & Lupton, 1996; Rose, 1996). For example, recent critical research examining harm minimisation has argued that the construction of the neo-liberal subject as an autonomous, rational and calculating agent fails to account for structural constraints on individual agency or how social and political responsibilities constrain agency (Fraser, 2004). Drawing on the work of Foucault, post-structuralists have been interested in *how* power has been applied or practised in a series of ongoing and multiple subjugations that operate within the social body rather than from above it (Armstrong, 1993; Foucault, 1990a; Lupton, 1995). Foucaultian criticism has focussed on the body as a site of power, examining ways in which unhealthy or at-risk bodies have been rendered productive and responsible through the strategic mobilisation of disciplinary health practices (Rose, 1994). Public health has as its locus the institutions and individuals of civil society. It might be described as a technology of everyday life in that it embeds social controls in the fabric of everyday interaction, rather than imposing them from above in the form of sovereign commands.

While social scientists have given ample attention to repressive functions of control, which we label here sanitationist practices, only recently has attention turned to more subtle practices of social control which we describe here as hygienist. Here we consider the relationship between the two, particularly how each might be embodied in one regime, namely, public health. In a similar way, Lupton (2014) has documented various modes of self-tracking, noting a tendency to present it merely as a form of participatory self-surveillance, juxtaposed to more covert or imposed forms of surveillance. She documents, for example, 'private' or 'communal' modes of self-tracking, as distinct from 'pushed' or 'imposed'. She further argues that self-tracking technologies have been dispersed into multiple domains, with evidence emerging of 'function creep' as private and participatory modes become collective and imposed (Lupton, 2014). This paper furthers this work by examining the relationship between these technologies of power. In particular, we are interested in how hygienist practices, which may include a range of self-governance technologies including self-management, self-monitoring and self-tracking, often play an important role in the social control of drug use.

Following the normalisation theory of illicit drug use, it is our contention that in contemporary Western contexts, drug use deemed to be 'recreational' is normalised as unremarkable, non-pathological and an intrinsic part of leisure culture, as opposed to being defined as a deviant or criminal activity requiring formal regulation (Measham & Shiner, 2009). While there is a continuing concern with drug use that is defined as problematic, Australian drug policy emphasises prevention, as encapsulated in the diverse social practices of harm reduction. In this context, the broader trend in Western societies towards crime prevention might be viewed as a neo-liberal response to the perceived failures of state responses to illicit drug use (Garland, 1997). Sovereign measures deployed in recent decades to address problems associated with illicit drug use have resulted in a growth of imprisonment among people who use drugs, particularly in the United States (MacCoun & Reuter, 2001). At the same time there have emerged developments which might best be described as new modes of governing illicit substances, each entailing new objectives, new criminological discourses and forms of practical knowledge and techniques of implementation (Rose, 1999; Seddon, 2007). Harm-reduction regimes embody diverse strategies of governance in which drug use may be posited not as a departure from rationalised conduct, explicable in terms of pathology or inadequate socialisation, but as continuous in normal social interaction and explicable by reference to standard motivational patterns. To this extent, what we term here hygienist practices of power have regulated drug use.

Public health strategies have sought to positively realise 'good health' by promoting long-term behavioural transformations in the subjects it has invested in. Self-tracking comprises a number of technologies, both digital and other, which assist in the creation of responsible, ethical, 'healthy' subjects. What distinguishes public health from other apparatuses of power, which have previously dealt with problems of disease control or health management, is the promotion of broader population health and well-being. Public health comprises multiple technologies of governance that typically require the collusion of those it seeks to invest in. What we describe below is not so much the techniques of self-governance, but how harm reduction operates to reconfigure those who use drugs as health conscious citizens, capable of rational actions and self-regulation. Health and hygiene are not simply abstract standards imposed upon people; rather health is an enactment of selfhood which people actively choose in their day-to-day practices.

Sanitationism and hygienicist practices of public health

Sanitationist practices are prohibitive, typically enforcing quarantine or a regime of treatment on the body through the intermittent deployment of practices of domination. Sanitationist strategies operate according to a binary mechanics of *difference*, which functions to isolate or separate polluted bodies from a moral community. Under contemporary Western regimes of public health, sanitationist practices have much symbolic force, power reinforcing the sovereign right of the state to provide security in the form of population health, in a given territory.

Sovereign practices of power might be said to 'leperise' sick or polluted bodies. Historically, the exclusion of the leper was neither an act of 'punishment' nor 'cure', but may best be understood as a symbolic action designed to communicate certain ideas about community (Clay, 1966). As a particular practice, sovereign power has declined in relevance since the seventeenth and eighteenth centuries, being a secondary feature of power relations rather than a principle mode of operation. In contemporary contexts, authoritative power, operating through sovereign practices, criminalises people who use drugs, articulates the 'addict' as Other – polluted and polluting – and imposes forms of self-tracking for surveillance purposes.

In contrast to, and to some degree, in tension with sanitationist practices, hygienist practices operate according to a principle of *differentiation*, which operates to connect, include and animate difference within the social. Rather than repress difference, hygienist practices might be said to have the strategic aim of empowering 'at-risk' bodies by providing protection, cure, reformation and rehabilitation. These measures have had the common purpose of 're-socialising' the body, or ensuring that it reaches a certain standard of sociality deemed medically and socially desirable. Hygienist practices function as technologies of the self, allowing for bodies to be regulated at a distance through the promotion of social norms and rights and responsibilities.

During the sixteenth and seventeenth centuries, there was a shift in the way in which government was understood and contemplated in Western Europe. This period marked the beginning of what can be described as the biopolitical age in which problems of population, such as sexual and reproductive hygiene, came to be interconnected with issues of national policy and power (Gordon, 1991). While medical knowledge was concerned with individual health, the emergence of a biopolitical collective enterprise of public health during the nineteenth century encompassed broad categories of the population and environment, including regulation of psychological, social and physical spheres of life (Petersen & Lupton, 1996, p. ix). The management of health was no longer just a matter of disciplining unhealthy bodies, but a complex system of health management that sought to guard the population as a whole.

Public health was largely made possible through the growth of statistical knowledge which enabled standards of normality to be calculated for population health, situating each individual in relation to it, and promoting and new ethics of the self (Osborne, 1996, pp. 104–105; Chadwick, 1965 [1842]). Government sought to foster individual lives in order to strengthen its own development, and health became an end in itself. The sovereign form of power which typically showed itself in the right to take life or leperise became overshadowed by a power that sought to maintain and develop life (Foucault, 1990a). This new disciplinary power sought to train, heal and cure the body, and to develop and produce life. The body become a principal site of health regulation and practices of life and technologies of health were developed to measure forms of conduct. Contemporary self-monitoring, self-management and self-tracking technologies may be described as disciplinary to the extent that individuals seek to learn more about the self in order to improve health.

According to Foucault the process of self-formation encompasses both a moral code and ethical practices (Rabinow, 1997, p. xxvi). Individuals conform to a moral code by simply obeying external forms of authority or governance without any mutual or reciprocal relationship, while ethical practices construct a relationship to oneself through techniques of everyday living (Kendall, 2011). Moral conduct not only brings individuals into conformity with dominant values and rules, but also into a mode of being through ethical practices of self-formation. The individual becomes both the object of their moral practices and an ethical subject of their moral goal (Foucault, 1985, 1997). This process of interaction between authority and the self is what Foucault called 'governmentality' (Foucault, 1997).

Contemporary drug use and public health

As the medical gaze widened from the individual body to the social body, epidemiology in public health policy came to be a way of viewing drug 'addiction' as a biopolitical problem (Berridge, 1999). There were growing anxieties about excessive opiate use for non-medical purposes, particularly among the lower classes and Chinese populations who were viewed as sources of unhealthy conditions and contagion. These concerns resulted in the enactment of a variety of Poisons Acts between the late nineteenth century and the 1930s in England, the United States and Australia to prohibit the use and sale of a range of substances (Berridge & Edwards, 1987; Manderson, 1993; Musto, 1999). The so-called addicts came to be variously represented in terms of their pathology (Valverde, 1998), their epidemiology (Robertson et al., 1986), and their productivity and functionality (Seddon, 2011). Binaries developed around drug use, emphasising legal and illegal forms of use, and categories of 'recreational' or 'addicted' forms of drug use. Strategies emerged in Western jurisdictions to manage health and social problems associated with drug use that was deemed to be pathological. Drug policies and strategies were not simply a way of reducing medical or social harms but were also a means of allowing the 'addict' to lead an economically productive and socially responsible life (Berridge, 1992, pp. 58–61).

By the 1980s fears of a global AIDS epidemic had prompted major drug policy shifts in Western contexts (Mold & Berridge, 2010, p. 109). The main concern of the HIV/AIDS epidemic for health professionals was the risk that the virus could spread from people who inject drugs to the wider population through sexual transmission (Robertson et al., 1986; Walmsley, 2012). Harm reduction subsequently became identified with HIV/AIDS prevention and also with addictions treatments which shifted from a focus on abstinence to an emphasis on harm minimisation (Roe, 2005). In Australia and the UK, community-based strategies such as needle syringe programs were developed to reduce the risk of people who used illicit drugs spreading HIV to the general population. These strategies brought people who used illicit drugs into services where they had access to harm-reduction information and injecting equipment (Mold

& Berridge, 2010, pp. 109–110). While there has been widespread political resistance to harm reduction, especially in the United States, where education has traditionally deployed scare tactics and an exaggerated dichotomy exists between legal and illegal drugs in order to mandate total abstinence, there have been signs that harm reduction is gaining policy ground (Gowan, Whetstone, & Andic, 2012).

The rationale of harm reduction is inclusive, to enable people who use drugs to minimise harm to themselves and the community by practising responsible, self-regulating, safe drug use. By utilising harm-reduction strategies, programs and techniques, people who use drugs are able to become active citizens in managing and monitoring their own risk (Dean, 1999, p. 168) and act as responsible consumers through hygienist, low-risk drug use practices (Seddon, 2010, p. 87).

In the past decade or so there has been a proliferation of technologies and devices for monitoring, managing and tracking people's activities, bodies and behaviours. These range from voluntarily collecting information on oneself to coercively imposing self-tracking devices upon individuals for surveillance or to monitor compliance through wearable devices (Lupton, 2014). This paper analyses these self-governance technologies in the context of contemporary drug use as a practice of the self that aligns with civic expectations of taking responsibility for managing and governing one's health according to an ethos of harm reduction.

This study finds that respondents voluntarily utilised harm reduction through self-monitoring and self-management technologies using dedicated websites designed to inform and reduce drug-related harms. These online communities of people who use drugs are able to compare drug experiences, and share harm-reduction information, such as data on 'safe' drug dosages and reports on 'good' and 'bad' ecstasy pills. These social networks encourage responsible drug use and peer learning, through sites such as Bluelight (http://www.bluelight.org/vb/content), Erowid (https://www.erowid.org) and ecstasydata.org (https://www.ecstasydata.org). Respondents also practised self-management to reduce harms associated with injecting drug use, and several participants reported the use of imposed self-surveillance technologies (Lupton, 2014) as part of broader criminal justice harm-reduction interventions. Although none of our respondents reported the use of digital self-tracking devices to monitor their drug use, in recent years there has been a proliferation of apps and other online networked, digital, technologies for self-tracking drug use have opened up new ways of 'doing harm reduction'. For example, Drugs Meter (www.drugsmeter.com) is an independent website which links to drugs meter apps for a range of illicit substances in addition to alcohol and tobacco. The apps provide comparative drug use data for people in similar geographic locations to determine the level of the user's drug use on a scale of lowest to highest. The apps also provide a comparative risk and harm analysis based on the user's current health status, habitual use of a substance and use of other substances. Another harm-reduction app, DrugLog, which is currently under development, is available via Google Play, and allows users to monitor their drug usage in order to create safer drug use (https://play.google.com/store/apps/details?id=lolbellum.druglog). Users are able to request a notification when their drug use reaches a nominated dose, or a reminder to stay safe, for example, by drinking water every 30 minutes.

Method

This study which was undertaken between 2011 and 2012 sought to better understand the biopolitical governance of drug use in contemporary contexts. Contemporary drug use is examined as a way to explore the interaction of authoritative power and technologies of the self in the formation of ethical subjects of harm reduction. Following ethics approval qualitative interviews were conducted with 29 people aged 18–25 years who used illicit drugs. Young people are the focus of the investigation because their drug use tends to be more diverse than older people, and therefore potentially provides richer material for the research (Australian Institute of Health and Welfare, 2011; Hammersley, Khan, & Ditton, 2002). Respondents reported that they used drugs on a regular basis, and for the purposes of the research, regular use was defined in terms of weekly to fortnightly use for a period of at least two months.

Young people interviewed for the research comprised 9 respondents who were regular users of a youth service in Brisbane, 16 students from three separate Brisbane universities, and 4 respondents who worked full-time. All interview respondents chose a pseudonym to protect their identity and these have been used in reporting of the results.

Respondents from the youth service used drugs on a daily basis and regularly injected drugs. Their preferred substances were the synthetic opioid oxycodone, amphetamines and heroin. These drugs were often substituted with, or used in combination with, cannabis, alcohol or prescription medications, particularly when the user's drug of choice was unavailable. Preferred prescription medications included Xanax, buprenorphine, methadone, diazepam and temazepam.

All the respondents from the youth service reported being unemployed and homeless or living in temporary accommodation. They had regular contact with the criminal justice system, and all respondents had been incarcerated in a juvenile detention centre or an adult prison on at least one occasion for drug-related offences. Several participants were on probation orders from the courts, or had been released from prison on parole at the time of interview. The youth service provided access to free, clean, injecting equipment and educational advice about safe injecting practices.

In contrast, students and full-time workers interviewed for the research reported their drug use as recreational and a temporary source of leisure or fun. None of them had ever been charged with a drug offence, and all had aspirations for a good career, domestic and family happiness and security. Most of these respondents ($n = 18$) regularly used ecstasy and cannabis, while four respondents used LSD and one student and one full-time worker regularly used amphetamines.

Interview data were coded and thematically analysed to capture the contexts of respondents' drug use, their concepts of harm and how their drug use was governed. Emergent themes were then grouped into concepts relating to Foucault's governmentality framework. This allowed for an investigation of how subjectivity is formed at the intersection of technologies of governance, and practices of drug use.[1]

This paper is not intended as an analysis of contemporary drug use or as an evaluation of contemporary drug policies. Rather, the research sought to understand how typologies of people who use drugs, such as 'addicts' and 'recreational drug users', form the basis of contemporary governance of illicit drug use, and translate into strategies of management of people who use drugs (O'Malley, 2004; O'Malley & Valverde, 2004; Vrecko, 2010). We also use the interview data to explore the power effects of these discourses and practices in order to understand how people who use drugs govern their own drug use through self-monitoring, self-management and self-tracking techniques.

Ethical self-governance of drug use practices

Students and workers interviewed for the research discussed their drug use in terms of responsibility, regulated pleasure and risk management. They regularly accessed drug networking sites and pill reports to share experiences and read information about the purity of their ecstasy pills. Danny, a 21-year-old worker in the entertainment industry, relied on data from online sources to responsibly manage his drug use:

> I'll always test it first to make sure I'm getting it from legitimate sources ... I do my research via Bluelight, which tell you what sort of ecstasy and acid is ok and what to look out for ... and erowid.org, the Wikipedia of drugs ... it comes back to responsible drug use ... drug use is about responsible choice. (Danny)

Similarly, Vicki, a 22-year-old journalism student, was able to make responsible, informed decisions about her ecstasy use, based on peers' experiences shared through online pill reports:

> Pill reports are a good way to know which ecstasy is good or not ... (Vicki)

Respondents who injected drugs did not report the use of technologies such as online social networking methods to monitor their drug use, yet they were committed to an ethos of harm reduction through hygienic, safe, injecting practices.

Chris, a 23-year-old man who frequently injected amphetamines, oxycodone and heroin, explained:

> I manage my drug use safely ... I use fresh needles and stuff ... I don't share needles ... I don't go stupid on it. (Chris)

Mack, a 19-year-old person who regularly injected oxycodone, stated:

> I always use clean syringes ... I'm pretty pedantic about it. (Mack)

Similar to the students and workers, respondents who injected drugs relied on peer learning via shared experiences to monitor their own safe drug use. Anne, a 21-year-old woman who had spent many years injecting oxycodone and living on the street, described herself as a peer educator:

> ... I want to be an example to them ... give advice to young people ... . I took a course ... so that I can be a peer educator about safe injecting and disposal ... all part and parcel of being a user ... and I have the authority to be able to educate these people on what they're doing wrong ... (Anne)

Mikki, a 23-year-old person who regularly injected oxycodone and heroin, explained that she educates less experienced people who use illicit drugs about safe injecting practices:

> ... it's good now because I teach young ones ... the bad things about drugs ... having dirty shots ... missing shots. (Mikki)

Anne's and Mikki's aspirations of self-improvement in order to help others illustrate how they form an ethical self through their own moral conduct and ethical practices, and their moral obligations to govern others in appropriate hygienist harm-reduction conduct. Anne and Mikki are then both the governed and the governor, monitoring and subjecting others who they educate in harm-reduction practices, while simultaneously monitoring and governing themselves (Foucault, 1990b; Kendall, 2011).

All respondents were scathing of those they perceived as undisciplined or irresponsible due to a failure to adequately self-monitor or exercise self-care in their drug use. Respondents who described their drug use as recreational expressed disgust for those who used drugs on a daily basis, or those who used methamphetamine or smoked marijuana in a bong rather than a joint. This was evident in comments by university students George, Jim and Vicki:

> People who use drugs all the time have no goals in life ... I have no respect for them ... you have to be responsible and know your limits. (George)
> Methamphetamine is disgusting and dirty ... the people are grubby ... the sort of people who become a junkie ... (Jim)
> ... only bogans smoke it [marijuana] in a dirty, disgusting bong ... they're lazy and unemployed ... or the school drop outs ... such as the apprentice tradies ... the ones that start smoking when they're at uni ... they're the social joint smokers. (Vicki)

Anne was intolerant of those she perceived to be dirty or irresponsible in their injecting drug use practices:

> ... dirty injecting makes you sick – why weren't they taught how to do it properly? ... I once saw a heroin junkie have a hit from an old can and he accidentally kicked dirt into it, but still shot it up ... that was so dirty ... .(Anne)

Respondents' comments illustrate how norms do not only establish binaries between users of illicit drugs and non-users, nor do they simply differentiate between problematic and regulated drug use. Rather, those whose drug use is deemed to be 'problematic' are actively differentiated according to collective norms of responsible usage and self-management (Simmonds & Coomber, 2009). Harm-reduction practices enacted through education, counselling, safe ecstasy use or safe injecting practices reproduce subjects who attribute a moral subjectivity to themselves, and aim to reform themselves according to its norms to achieve self-optimisation (Pereira & Carrington, 2015; Rose, 1996).

Transforming people who use drug into ethical citizens

We have seen how disciplinary power operates in through hygienist public health strategies to produce healthy, responsible citizens. Communal self-monitoring and self-management techniques such as sharing drug experiences, data on appropriate dosages, and knowledge of safe pills or safe injecting techniques are practices of selfhood which conform to social and civic expectations concerning responsibly governing one's drug use to improve life chances (Lupton, 2014). We turn now to the regulation of people who use drugs through sanitationist controls which operate at the intersection of public health and criminal justice as extra-judicial functions. In this context we explore the use of coercive or imposed surveillance and self-tracking technologies to understand how those who use drugs in ways that are defined as problematic are often perceived as unwilling or unable to reconstruct their subjectivity in line with moral citizenship. They are subjected to reformative technologies of governance so they might act on themselves to become responsible, functioning citizens.

In contemporary societies there is an expectation that people who use illicit drugs take responsibility for their own conduct and its consequences, and ensure their own reformation to enable their participation in ethical citizenship and membership of the moral community (Rose, 1999, 2000). People who use drugs are subsequently encouraged to become active collaborators working with healthcare professionals, rather than passive recipients of care (Moore & Fraser, 2006).

Those who are deemed unwilling to utilise appropriate resources and take precautions against illness, or are unwilling or unable to take public health advice to enable participatory citizenship may be constructed as either pathological or criminal. They may also be presented as 'dirty' and generally asocial among peers, or sociopathic or psychopathic within professional assessments. Recalcitrant populations such as repeat drug offenders may be subjected to imposed surveillance and self-tracking technologies which are tied to incarceration, such as compulsory detox or rehabilitation programs, and expanded penal sanctions, such as tightly sanctioned probation and parole conditions (Lupton, 2014; Vrecko, 2010). Although these extra-judicial programs have sometimes been perceived as 'soft' options that replace harsher punishments such as incarceration, in reality they are frequently governed by tight surveillance and regulation, and can result in lengthy prison sentences for those who fail to comply (Rose, 1999, 2000; Vrecko, 2010).

These extra-judicial programs usually encompass both hygienist and sanitationist forms of governance. It may be argued that there is an inherent tension in such programs because law enforcement is fundamentally at odds with harm-reduction principles (Miller, 2001; Roe, 2005). For example, tighter levels of scrutiny and surveillance for participants of drug treatment and rehabilitation programs have been justified on the basis of harm-reduction principles. In order to stem the flow of illicit drugs in prisons, prisoners are frequently required to undergo urinalysis, strip searches and internal body cavity searches. Although these detection techniques are justified on the basis of minimising the 'harm caused by drugs to staff, offenders and society in general' (Queensland Corrective Services, 2006; Queensland Corrective Services, 2015a, 2015b), they often have the effect of net-widening or expanding criminal sanctions.

All of our study participants recruited from the youth service had at some stage been subjected to sanitationist controls through the use of imposed surveillance and tracking techniques. Although no participants reported the use of digital monitoring devices or biometric self-tracking devices, these types of technologies are an intrinsic part of Queensland Corrective Services' offender management programs (Queensland Corrective Services, 2015a, 2015b). Several participants described their experiences of imposed compulsory, regular urine testing, mandatory 12-step programs, and coercive drug rehabilitation programs inside prison, or as part of their parole or probation conditions following release from prison. Failure to complete rehabilitation programs or provide clean drug-free urine samples could result in further court processes and often a period of incarceration.

Chris, a 22-year-old man and repeat drug offender who had injected amphetamines for several years, described his experience of compulsory drug rehabilitation:

I got put into rehab after gaol ... the judge sent me there ... now I have to go back to gaol because I took off from rehab ... the first thing I did was go for some dope. (Chris)

Roscoe, a 22-year-old homeless man, described his experiences of a medicated drug detoxification in prison. He started attending Narcotics Anonymous in prison and continued to attend while on probation following his release. Roscoe's probation conditions included urine testing and he expected to return to prison in the near future due to a 'dirty urine' test:

When I first went to gaol I was put in the Drug Unit ... it was a three-month course ... we were all put on Valium in the morning and night ... now they got me doing urines and stuff for my parole ... in gaol I started doing an NA twelve steps course ... but I don't keep going because I had a dirty urine last week, so now I'll go back to gaol. (Roscoe)

Chuck, a 23-year-old man who had used amphetamines and heroin, had spent four years in gaol. He described his strict parole conditions involving frequent drug urine testing:

I'm on parole for two years ... I have to give three clean urines a week ... I already had a dirty urine so I'm expecting do another two years. (Chuck)

Reformative, self-regulating technologies such as 12-step programs and mandatory rehabilitation for repeat drug offenders encourage those who use drugs like Chris, Roscoe and Chuck, to transform themselves into citizens (Rose, 1999, pp. 271–273). These imposed and coercive forms of governance assume an alignment between the interests of people who use illicit drugs and the governing interests of authorities (Garland, 1997).

Those who are labelled as 'recalcitrant' like Chris, Roscoe and Chuck are identified for coercive treatment due to their unwillingness or inability to reconstruct their subjectivity in line with reformers' goals of self-empowerment and active moral citizenship (Garland, 1997; Rose, 1996). They have subsequently been regulated by sanitationist controls using an ensemble of surveillance and tracking practices and technologies, in order to maintain normative boundaries. They have also been subjected to hygienist public health and educational initiatives, which have focussed upon specific communities to 'empower' them so that they might develop certain skills to help them exercise greater regulation and control over their lives (Kinsman, 1996). Ethics of subjectivity are linked to procedures of power, and for 'problem' populations such as Chris, Roscoe and Chuck, power is tied to coercive technologies of reformation (Cruikshank, 1993; Rose, 1996). They are 'obliged' to engage with their own freedom by 'choosing' to pursue self-fulfilment, in line with reformers' goals of rehabilitation, and the broader objectives of government (Rose, 2000; Rose & Miller, 1992).

Concluding comments

Public health might be considered as a historically specific initiative designed to resolve or manage a number of biopolitical problems, including drug use. It incorporates elements of ethical and policing strategies to health, the imperative of health being achieved through the mobilisation of practices of the self and practices of domination. Contemporary harm-reduction programs deploy both sanitationist and hygienist technologies in the governance of injecting drug use. Harm-reduction regimes have not marked a reduction in the operations of power, but have signalled a change in the way in which power is operationalised and practised. Older practices of power have not simply vanished or become inoperative, but have been co-opted into the operation of contemporary governmental apparatuses.

This process of governing operates within the social body of people who use illicit drugs, through self-governance involving self-management, self-monitoring, surveillance and self-tracking techniques. Public health, as a regime of power, governs people who use illicit drugs, but this is not a repressive top-down form of power, and does not necessarily imply a violation of the interests of people who use illicit drugs. Rather, the user actively participates in their own governance through reformist technologies that are embedded in public health policies, specifically harm-reduction programs. This is illustrated in respondents' descriptions of their ethics of responsible, disciplined drug use, their safe injecting and their condemnation of those deemed to be 'dirty' or unhygienic on account of the failure to comply with the moral authority of harm reduction. Public health as a regime of power does not so much create difference as it does differentiation. People who use illicit drugs are taught to behave in ways that prevent or minimise potential harm to the social body. Failure to do so has come to signal social and individual irresponsibility. As shown here, people who use illicit drugs understand the self and other people who use illicit drugs in relation to norms of good health, responsibility and functionality, which are achieved through ethical drug use. The objective of power is not to leperise the people who use illicit drugs, but to reintegrate them into the social.

As we have illustrated, recalcitrant populations such as repeat drug offenders have been governed through sanitationist controls such as incarceration and mandatory rehabilitation in order to promote and maintain normative boundaries. Using self-governing technologies of self-management, self-monitoring, imposed surveillance and digital self-tracking technologies they are also subjected to hygienist initiatives such as extra-judicial programs, so they might act on themselves, by 'choosing' personal goals of self-improvement that are aligned with governmental objectives. These 'empowering' initiatives oblige people who use illicit drugs to engage in their own freedom through ethical practices of responsible management and regulation of their drug use in order that they might become productive, functioning citizens. Public health operates according to a principle of exposure, so that it is not only the sovereign's eyes that are permitted to see and watch, but all persons watch each other, as the governed and the governor, in order that they might better see and know themselves.

Note

1. In this paper we use the term 'illicit' to describe the use of illegal substances, or the use of legal substances in ways other than that which is intended or prescribed. We also use the terms 'addict' and 'recreational' in places where respondents identified as such or where we are describing an historical concept of drug use. We acknowledge that the concepts of addiction and recreational drug use are complex and contested, and references to 'addicts', 'addiction' or 'recreational drug use' in this paper are in no way intended to describe the characteristics of the respondents.

Disclosure statement

No potential conflict of interest was reported by the authors.

References

Adkins, L. (2001). Risk, culture, self-reflexivity and the making of sexual hierarchies. *Body and Society, 7*(1), 35–55.

Armstrong, D. (1993). Public health spaces and the fabrication of identity. *Sociology, 27*, 393–410.

Australian Institute of Health and Welfare. (2011). *2010 National drug strategy household survey report, drug statistics series* (Number 25, Cat. No. PHE 145). Canberra: Australian Institute of Health and Welfare. Retrieved from Australian Institute of Health and Welfare: http://www.aihw.gov.au/publication-detail/?id=32212254712

Berridge, V. (1992). Harm minimization and public health: An historical perspective. In N. Heather, A. Wodak, E. Nadelmann, & P. O'Hare (Eds.), *Psychoactive drugs and harm reduction: From faith to science London* (pp. 55–64). London: Whurr Publishers.

Berridge, V. (1999). *Opium and the people: Opiate use and drug control policy in the nineteenth and early twentieth century England*. London: Free Association Books.

Berridge, V., & Edwards, G. (1987). *Opium and the people: Opiate use in nineteenth-century England*. London: Yale University Press.

Chadwick, E. (1965 [1842]). *Report on the sanitary condition of the labouring population of Great Britain*. Edinburgh: Edinburgh University Press.

Clay, R. M. (1966). *The medieval hospitals of England*. London: Frank Cass.

Cruikshank, B. (1993). Revolutions within: Self-government and self-esteem. In A. Barry, T. Osborne, & N. Rose (Eds.), *Foucault and political reason: Liberalism, neo-liberalism and rationalities of government* (pp. 231–252). London: UCL Press.

Dean, M. (1999). *Governmentality: Power and rule in modern society*. London: Sage Publications.

Foucault, M. (1985). *The history of sexuality, volume 2: The use of pleasure*. Translated by Robert Hurley. New York, NY: Random House.

Foucault, M. (1990a). *The history of sexuality, volume 1: An introduction*. New York, NY: Random House.

Foucault, M. (1990b). *The use of pleasure: Volume 2 of the history of sexuality*. Translated by Robert Hurley. New York, NY: Vintage Books.

Foucault, M. (1997). The ethics of the concern for self as a practice of freedom. In P. Rabinow, & M. Foucault (Eds.), *Ethics, subjectivity and truth: The essential works of Michel Foucault 1954–1984, volume one* (pp. 281–302). New York, NY: The New Press.

Fraser, S. (2004). "It's your life!": Injecting drug users, individual responsibility and hepatitis C prevention'. *Health: An International Journal for the Social Study of Health, Illness and Medicine, 8*(2), 199–221.

Garland, D. (1997). Governmentality and the problem of crime: Foucault, criminology, sociology. *Theoretical Criminology, 1*(2), 173–214.

Gordon, C. (1991). Governmental rationality: An introduction. In G. Burchall, C. Gordon, & P. Miller (Eds.), *The Foucault effect: Studies in governmentality* (pp. 1–52). Chicago: University of Chicago Press.

Gowan, T., Whetstone, S., & Andic, T. (2012). Addiction, agency, and the politics of self-control: Doing harm reduction in a heroin users' group. *Social Science & Medicine, 74*, 1251–1260.

Hammersley, R., Khan, F., & Ditton, J. (2002). Ecstasy and the rise of the chemical generation. *International Journal of Drug Policy, 13*(5), 437–438.

Kendall, G. (2011). Foucaultian approaches to the self. In A. Elliott (Ed.), *The Routledge handbook of identity studies* (pp. 67–82). London: Routledge.

Kinsman, G. (1996). 'Responsibility' as a strategy of governance: Regulating people living with AIDS and lesbians and gay men in Ontario. *Economy and Society, 25*, 393–409.

Lupton, D. (1995). *The imperative of health: Public health and the regulated body*. London: Sage.

Lupton, D. (2013). Quantifying the body: Monitoring and measuring health in the age of health technologies. *Critical Public Health, 23*(4), 393–403.

Lupton, D. (2014). *Self-tracking modes: Reflexive self-monitoring and data practices*. Paper presented at the Imminent Citizens: Personhood and Identity Politics in the Informatic Age workshop, 27 August, ANU: Canberra. Retrieved from Social Science Research Network: http://papers.ssrn.com/sol3/papers.cfm?abstract_id=2483549

Lupton, D. (2015). Quantified sex: A critical analysis of sexual and reproductive self-tracking using apps. *Culture, Health & Sexuality, 17*(4), 440–453.

MacCoun, R., & Reuter, P. (2001). *Drug war heresies: Learning from other vices, times and places*. Cambridge: Cambridge University Press.

Manderson, D. (1993). *From Mr Sin to Mr Big: A history of Australian drug laws*. Melbourne: Oxford University Press.

Measham, F., & Shiner, M. (2009). The legacy of 'normalisation': The role of classical and contemporary criminological theory in understanding young people's drug use. *International Journal of Drug Policy, 20*, 502–508.

Miller, P. (2001). A critical review of the harm minimization ideology in Australia. *Critical Public Health, 11*(2), 167–178.

Mold, A., & Berridge, V. (2010). *Voluntary action and illegal drugs: Health and society in Britain since the 1960s*. London: Palgrave Macmillan.

Moore, D., & Fraser, S. (2006). Putting at risk what we know: Reflecting on the drug-using subject in harm reduction and its political implications. *Social Science & Medicine, 62*, 3035–3047.

Musto, D. (1999). *The American disease: Origins of narcotics control*. Oxford: Oxford University Press.

Nettleton, S. (1997). Governing the risk self: How to become healthy, wealthy and wise. In A. Petersen, & R. Bunton (Eds.), *Foucault, health and medicine* (pp. 207–222). London: Routledge.

O'Malley, P. (2004). Risking drug use. In P. O'Malley (Ed.), *Risk, uncertainty and government* (pp. 155–172). London: Glass House Press.

O'Malley, P., & Valverde, M. (2004). Pleasure, freedom and drugs: The uses of 'pleasure' in liberal governance on drug and alcohol consumption. *Sociology, 38*(1), 25–42.

Osborne, T. (1996). Security and vitality: Drains, liberalism and power in the nineteenth century. In A. Barry, T. Osborne, & N. Rose (Eds.), *Foucault and political reason: Liberalism, neo-liberalism and rationalities of government* (pp. 99–122). London: UCL Press.

Patron, C., Hansen, M., Fernandez-Luque, L., & Lau, A. (2012). *Self-tracking, social media and personal health records for patient empowered self-care*. University of San Francisco Scholarship Repository, Nursing and Health Professions Faculty Research, Research Paper 17. Retrieved from University of San Francisco Scholarship Repository: http://repository.usfca.edu/cgi/viewcontent.cgi?article=1016&context=nursing_fac

Pereira, M., & Carrington, K. (2015). Irrational addicts and responsible pleasure seekers: Constructions of the drug user. *Critical Criminology*. doi:10.1007/s10612-015-9298-z

Petersen, A., & Lupton, D. (1996). *The new public health: Health and self in the age of risk*. St Leonards: Allen and Unwin.

Queensland Corrective Services. (2006). *Drug strategy 2006: Tackling drug abuse and addiction, changing lives in Queensland prisons*. Brisbane: Queensland Corrective Services, Brisbane. Retrieved from Queensland Corrective Services: http://www.correctiveservices.qld.gov.au/Resources/Policies/Documents/DrugStrategy.pdf

Queensland Corrective Services. (2015a). *Procedure – Substance testing – Corrective services facilities – Random and targeted*. Brisbane: Queensland Corrective Services. Retrieved from Queensland Corrective Services: http://www.correctiveservices.qld.gov.au/Resources/Procedures/Offender_Management/documents/ofmprosubtstrantar.shtml

Queensland Corrective Services. (2015b). *Electronic monitoring*. Brisbane: Queensland Corrective Services. Retrieved from Queensland Corrective Services: http://www.correctiveservices.qld.gov.au/About_Us/The_Department/Probation_and_Parole/Electronic_Monitoring/index.shtml

Rabinow, P. (1997). Introduction: The history of systems of thought. In P. Rabinow (Ed.), *Ethics, subjectivity and truth: The essential works of Michel Foucault 1954–1984, volume one,* (pp. xi–xlv). New York, NY: The New Press.

Robertson, J., Bucknall, A., Welsby, P., Roberts, J., Inglis, J., Peutherer, J., & Brettle, R. (1986). Epidemic of AIDS related virus (HTLV-III/LAV) infection among intravenous drug abusers. *British Medical Journal, 292*, 527–529.

Roe, G. (2005). Harm reduction as paradigm: Is better than bad good enough? The origins of harm reduction. *Critical Public Health, 15*(3), 243–250.

Rose, N. (1994). Medicine, history and the present. In C. Jones, & R. Porter (Eds.), *Reassessing Foucault: Power, medicine and the body* (pp. 48–72). London: Routledge.

Rose, N. (1996). *Inventing our selves: Psychology, power and personhood.* Cambridge: Cambridge University Press.

Rose, N. (1999). *Powers of freedom: Reframing political thought.* Cambridge: Cambridge University Press.

Rose, N. (2000). Government and control. *British Journal of Criminology, 40,* 321–339.

Rose, N., & Miller, P. (1992). Political power beyond the state: Problematics of government. *The British Journal of Criminology, 43*(2), 173–205.

Seddon, T. (2007). Coerced drug treatment in the criminal justice system: Conceptual, ethical and criminological issues. *Criminology and Criminal Justice, 7*(3), 269–286.

Seddon, T. (2010). *A history of drugs: Drugs and freedom in the liberal age.* Abington: Routledge.

Seddon, T. (2011). What is a problem drug user? *Addiction, Research and Theory, 19*(4), 334–343.

Simmonds, L., & Coomber, R. (2009). Injecting drug users: A stigmatised and stigmatising population. *International Journal of Drug Policy, 20,* 121–130.

Swan, M. (2012). Health 2050: The realization of personalized medicine through crowdsourcing, the quantified self, and the participatory biocitizen. *Journal of Personalized Medicine, 2,* 93–118.

Swan, M. (2013). The quantified self: Fundamental disruption in Big data science and biological discovery. *Big Data, 1*(2), 85–99.

Valverde, M. (1998). *Diseases of the will: Alcohol and the dilemmas of freedom.* Cambridge: Cambridge University Press.

Vrecko, S. (2010). Civilizing technologies and the control of deviance. *BioSocieties, 5*(1), 36–51.

Walmsley, I. (2012). Governing the injecting drug user: Beyond needle fixation. *History of the Human Sciences, 25*(4), 90–107.

Mobile, wearable and ingestible health technologies: towards a critical research agenda

Emma Rich and Andy Miah

ABSTRACT

In this article, we review critical research on mobile and wearable health technologies focused on the promotion of 'healthy lifestyles'. We begin by discussing key governmental and policy interests which indicate a shift towards greater digital integration in health care. Subsequently, we review relevant research literature, which highlights concerns about inclusion, social justice, and ownership of mobile health data, which we argue, provoke a series of key sociological questions that are in need of additional investigation. We examine the expansion of what counts as health data, as a basis for advocating the need for greater research into this area. Finally, we consider how digital devices raise questions about the reconfiguration of relationships, behaviours, and concepts of individuality.

Introduction

In present times, the growth of mobile and wearable technologies is radically reconfiguring health care, as they allow people to self-monitor and regulate their health practices, often without the involvement of any healthcare professional. For example, wristbands fitted with motions sensors use algorithms to track everyday activities, such as walking or hours slept. The global significance of these transformations is vast, as mHealth activity is capable of functioning in environments where there is a limited technological infrastructure. Thus, exploring the potential of mHealth is fast becoming a global priority, especially where resources are limited and where more people have access to a mobile device than a hospital or clinic. While there is much to celebrate about the transformative capacity of mHealth, there is also a more critical discourse emerging in response to what Lupton (2014a, p. 706) describes as the 'prevailing solutionist and instrumental approaches to the application of digital technologies to medicine and public health'.

Extending the critical analysis of mHealth, we examine consumer-oriented technologies that are pertinent to promoting healthy lifestyle behaviours, such as physical activity, body weight management, and food consumption. Wider concerns about the absence of regulation around such lifestyle apps underpin our interest in these categories of mHealth technologies (Powell, Landman, & Bates, 2014). Over 70% of all health apps fit into this category (Research2Guidance, 2014), but the expansion of health-related data reveals a much bigger picture of unregulated health apps. Our intention for this paper is to present an overview of critical digital health studies focused on these technologies and to signpost future research agendas. Our analysis begins with a review of the term mHealth, so as to establish the parameters of this field. We then focus on some of the recent notable contributions to the critical analysis of mHealth, examining the theoretical developments informing these analyses and exploring some of the challenges and emerging issues. Many of these wearable technologies and apps deserve individual empirical exploration – perhaps even the development of what might be termed *device ethnography* – though we focus on broad characteristics of these apps and the kinds of practices that occur within them. These insights indicate how the sociology of digital health, as a distinct research field, is in need of new methodological approaches, and cannot rely simply on established techniques.

Mhealth as a public health solution

Striving for technological efficiencies has long since been part of health care's internal logic. As such, the recent trend towards adopting mobile health tracking technology must be understood within the wider economics of care, which tend towards streamlining structures, systems, and resources. Increasingly, governments and health agencies treat mHealth as a way to deliver a more efficient and effective healthcare system. For example, in 2014, the British Government's vision statement for transforming health care in the face of a growing budget deficit announces that it will develop an 'expanding set of NHS accredited health apps that patients will be able to use to organise and manage their own health and care' (NHS England, 2014, p. 32). For the UK, it is perhaps the clearest indication of how the mobile device ecosystem will become a bigger part of how health care is managed. The rising appeal of digital health solutions to influence individual behaviours is therefore rationalized 'against the backdrop of contemporary public health challenges that include increasing costs, worsening outcomes, "diabesity" epidemics, and anticipated physician shortages' (Swan, 2012, p. 93). Policy investments in digital health care are justified based on their ability to deliver greater efficiency of overburdened healthcare systems. In terms of how health care is practiced, it therefore reflects a 'logic of choice' (Mol, 2008) whereby the concept of the patient as a customer or citizen emerges, along with the instrumental aspirations of digital interventions that transfer responsibility away from the state and onto the individual, an approach which, as many of the studies below indicate, aligns with neoliberal health perspectives. Governments and health organisations recognise the opportunities – and additional responsibilities – afforded by these technologies, as a means of delivering more effective healthcare systems (European Commission, 2010) and as a way of fostering a 'digitally engaged patient' (Lupton, 2013a).

The ubiquity of mobile devices, combined with the app ecosystem, has secured their place as a core driver of preventive health medicine, now recognised as 'mHealth' (Lupton, 2012; WHO, 2011). According to the WHO (2011), mHealth includes 'medical and public health practice supported by mobile devices, such as mobile phones, patient monitoring devices, personal digital assistants, and other wireless devices' and is a major growth area within health. In these new territories of health engagement, there is a growing market in mobile health apps categorised as 'lifestyle apps', and it is this category of mHealth technology to which we turn our attention. Focused on the promotion of healthy lifestyles, users can use these apps to track their exercise behaviour, body weight, and food consumption and they are the most downloaded health apps across mobile devices (Fox & Duggan, 2013). Such is their growing popularity and use that Google announced 2014 as the year of health and fitness apps (Boxall, 2014), recording this as their fastest-growing app category. Research2Guidance (2014) reinforces this claim, identifying health and fitness as the largest of all mHealth categories, with around 30% of the total share. Furthermore, Ruckenstein (2014, p. 68) observes that 'smart phones and tracking device have created a field of personal analytics and self-monitoring practices'. Within such environments, users learn how to look after themselves via the disciplining regularity of the device's presence, with its regular notifications, which encourage attentiveness to good behaviour, a trend that has been termed 'nag technology' in popular culture. The proliferation of wearable technologies, such as fitness bands and smart watches, enables this growth in self-monitoring by logging a user's movements and behaviours. In doing so, these devices record and track such details as body mass index, calories burnt, heart rate, physical activity patterns.

The rapid development of new technologies, their modes of organising data on bodies and the use of collective 'big data' demand the development of new theoretical approaches and methods. Health data produced both inside and outside of medical sites challenge the norms within different contexts of health and wellness, disrupting previously defined distinctions between patient and consumer, device and data, and health care and personal wellness. As such, it is no surprise that sociologists are turning to studies of health interactions in digital environments, as mobile and wearable technologies become a feature of everyday life. Indeed, the end point of this trend seems likely to be the emergence of ingestible sensors – or ingestibles – of which the first was granted United States Food and Drug Administration (FDA)approval for Proteus technologies in 2015 (Proteus, 2015). These trends raise questions about the adequacy of theoretical frameworks and methods for understanding mobile and wearable health technologies, questions which are at the core of our review of existing literature.

Quantify and know thy post human self: self-tracking and the quantified self

A number of studies examine a series of deeper trajectories that underpin the development of mHealth technology and the kinds of self-tracking behaviours that they nurture. For example, Henderson and Petersen (2002) describe processes of health and medical consumerism, where self-tracking technologies are encouraged so as to offer market solutions to health problems. In these cases, users purchase apps that capture data about their bodies which are designed to help them make more informed decisions about their health. An initial basis for interrogating such processes is found when considering the shift towards personalisation and individualisation of health care through such self-tracking technologies. Indeed, Foucault's concept of biopower is helpful here, as self-tracking and self-regulating through mHealth can be articulated as processes by which subjects engage in 'technologies of the self' (Foucault, 1988) to adhere to discourses of normalisation of the body.

Crucially, health practices are rendered visible through capturing body data in mHealth environments, which is transformed into a meaningful bodily classification, which denotes worth in terms of achievement, further reflecting the processes of biopower (Foucault, 1988). Consequently, Ruckenstein (2014) suggests that this form of 'personal analytics' is necessarily tied to notions of control and governmentality. Within this framework, health becomes the responsibility of the citizen as a productive consumer, whereby they become primarily responsible for their own health. To understand this more, authors are turning to theoretical concepts of pedagogy to explain how this form of biopower operates. For example, Williamson (2015 p. 140) investigates how self-tracking technologies are framed as 'biopedagogies of optimization' (Williamson, 2015, p. 140) through which 'self-quantification represents a new algorithmically mediated pedagogic technique for governing and ordering the body'. Elsewhere, Rich and Miah (2014) examine the public pedagogies of mHealth, calling for more research into understanding what and how people learn about their bodies and health through self-tracking and quantification. These sociological approaches reveal the impact of mHealth technologies on people's subjectivities and bodies, often in ways that are cause for concern.

More recently, new modes of quantifying the body and capturing data have prompted debates about ontological assumptions made about how bodies are experienced and rendered knowable. For instance, Ruckenstein (2014, p. 71) suggests that 'self-tracking tools abstract human bodies and minds into data flows that can be used and reflected upon' (Ruckenstein, 2014, p. 71). This work reveals processes of 'datafication of the body' (Mayer-Schönberger & Cukier, 2013, p. 48) where users are prompted to explore their datafied self, as a 'data double' (Haggerty & Ericson, 2000; Ruckenstein, 2014) so as to acquire knowledge of their bodies and purposefully monitor and regulate their health and body practices in line with related norms. As such, a body of work has focused on the way the body is being rendered knowable (Gilmore, 2015; Millington, 2015) through numbers, or as Gilmore (2015, p. 3) phrases it 'adding increasingly quantifiable means of accounting for one's being in the world'. Such work reveals how mHealth converges with neoliberal strategies of governance by promoting autonomous, enterprising individuals who are encouraged to capture data, share, analyse, and reflect on it in relation to data norms. A number of authors describe how the body becomes knowable as an object of quantified knowledge, reflecting a 'techo-utopian' view of the body (Lupton, 2014a). Increasingly, mHealth is therefore positioned as a route to 'self-betterment' or 'self-optimization' (Ruckenstein, 2014, p. 69) whereby it is not enough to 'have a more transparent view of oneself' but where 'one needs to respond to that knowledge and raise one's goals'. Thus, mHealth lifestyle technologies emphasise our ability to enhance one's physical or mental capacities, orienting individuals towards practices of monitoring, in pursuit of 'wellness' (Fries, 2008). In doing so, this neoliberal logic of the knowable body is part of a broader culture of risk management demarcating a shift towards 'post human optimisation' (Millington, 2015).

The wider sociology of health literature has considered the relationship between consumption and health (Fries, 2008) but is extended through the consideration of mHealth technologies, which prompt new questions about our understandings of 'humanness' and the relationship between the body and technology (Lupton, 2014b; Miah & Rich, 2008; Millington, 2015). Indeed, wearable technologies are rapidly being characterised as having distinct features which change our relationship to technology (Alrige & Chatterjee,

2015), which include their relative autonomy in how they can seamlessly capture data about our health. Also, these tracking technologies are now integrated into mobile operating systems, including Apple, with its built-in *Health Kit*, or Samsung with its *S Health* environment, which are key indications of how users must opt out, rather than opt in to biomonitoring. In each of these cases, the device comes pre-loaded with the requisite tracking technology. While one can switch off the tracking function, the default position upon purchase is for it to be active, reinforcing what we described earlier as the neo-liberal desire to be good citizens and monitor how we are doing. Drawing on the analytical work of Galloway (2004) of 'everyware' technologies, Gilmore (2015) develops the concept of 'everywear' technologies, described as those 'wearable' technologies, specifically within the fitness industry that reflect the ubiquitous technologies, 'tethered to bodies and, through habitualization, designed to add value to everyday life in the form of physical well-being' (Gilmore, 2015, p. 2) Elsewhere, in his critical examination of wearable posture-tracking technologies, Millington (2015) observes that 'new posture technologies trade optic for haptic surveillance. Sensors replace the eye with the touch en route to amassing extensive data on where posture goes "right" and "wrong". Through their ubiquity and automatic generation of data, he argues, 'surveillance is "passivised" as users do not so much participate as they do generate' (Millington, 2015, p. 6).

Such studies and the widespread use of these 'everywear' (Gilmore, 2015) technologies raises a series of questions about the autonomy of the device itself, reflecting a broader shift towards the 'sensor society' (Andrejevic & Burdon, 2015). No longer is it necessary to take out a device, open it up, turn it on, and navigate to the information we seek. Instead, the occupation of the device on our person, within our sensorial environment, allows it to function as if it were part of our body. Rich and Miah (2014, p. 308) describe this as 'posthuman technological mediation and prostheticisation', through which 'new sensorial experiences, such as the wearing of fitbit health bands, which vibrate when you achieve your activity goals, combine different pedagogical forces to produce embodied ways of knowing'.

Alongside this is the development of the *internet of things* – which describes a world where all objects are connected to the Internet. Presently, the approach to mHealth is centred mostly on the person (user) – their body literally. Yet, it is likely that an individual's body will become just one unit in a wider connected system, as captured in the work of Williamson (2015, p. 147) who suggests that 'rather than the cyborg image of the artificially prosthetized body, self-tracking connects bodies into a web of data, analytics and algorithmic forms of power – a "corporealgorithmic" coupling of bodies and flows of data'. These developments require theoretical approaches that can explore not only the relationship between sensory experiences and technology, but also 'the sociocultural constructs that also affect bodies materially' (Fox, 2016, p. 67):

> New materialism's relational and 'flat' ontology (in common with post-structuralism) eschews any notions of social structures, systems or mechanisms that can 'explain' social action and interactions. Instead, it explores the world and human lives by exploring how natural and cultural relations assemble, the forces (affects) between them and the capacities these affects produce. (Fox, 2016, p. 70)

On this view, whilst constructionist and post-structuralist approaches to mHealth may reveal important insights about the power and constitution of the subject of quantification, 'new materialisms' focused on 'matter and the materiality of social production' (Fox, 2016, p. 67) can provide new insights into pressing questions about mHealth. For example, how does the quantified, self-optimised body 'affect' other bodies (Deleuze, 1988), such as those in schools or in the workplace? How does rendering the body knowable through quantification impact upon the body's capacity? How does the sensorial experience of wearing technology shape what the body feels like and what it can do? As the body's capacity becomes knowable through quantification, what is the capacity for it to form relations with other bodies? How do such relationalities shape our understandings of relationships in health, such as those of the patient–professional? From this perspective, Fox (2011, p. 366) argues that health can be understood as the 'proliferation of a body's capacities to affect and be affected'. In other words, whilst it is important to understand what quantified bodies come to represent, the ontological orientation of new materialism or sociomaterialism provokes questions about what the body can *do* to other bodies in assemblages of quantification.

Critical questions on mhealth, big data, and the consumerism of health

The consequences of this biopolitics of mHealth, as outlined above, are only just beginning to be understood. A specific feature of mHealth applications and the data they generate is the capacity for that data to be shared with others, for example, within social media networks. There is a pressing need to address the public facing imposition of the mHealth industry, exacerbated by this 'sharing economy' (Barta & Neff, 2016) in which smart device users operate, as some fundamental assumptions about our lives are brought into question, such as the erosion of the public/private divide. To this end, mHealth does not simply respond to a vision of health, but can also be considered characteristic of a – 'confessional society' (Bauman, 2007). With their accompanying processes of surveillance and evaluation, these technologies imply certain, learned expectations of control, which are to be publicly displayed for evaluation by others as part of a process of 'lateral surveillance' (Andrejevic, 2005). Thus, to draw on the example of the popular running app 'Runtastic', the act of sharing the route, time, and distance of one's run, while being monitored by Runtastic, becomes a matter of shared knowledge, a matter of public dissemination or declaration, rather than of private record.

Apps and wearable devices can produce digital data on various bodily functions. Such data are not only shared via social media, but also form part of a broader 'digital data economy' (Lupton, 2013b, p. 30) which engages the interests of companies and health organisations. As designers continue to develop the digital market for health with new interfaces, critical digital health studies will need to address crucial issues concerning institutional use of data. This is a pertinent issue especially since users operate at a very individualistic level, without much sense of how their broader community is being exploited. To that end, we concur with Till (2014) that the emphasis within the sociology on digital self-tracking on the individualistic level must be expanded to consider how surveillance, subjectivity and the relationship to the self and body have wider implications. Researchers must consider such issues as how corporations manage (our) data and how they develop processes of digitisation and quantification.

Some authors are beginning to reveal the sociocultural implications of data mining and the collection of data on users that is used for marketing and other purposes (Lupton,

2014b; Till, 2014). Yet, we argue that there are many other questions to address. For instance, future studies of mHealth will find synergies with the studies of leisure sociology, in terms of the blurring of boundaries between work and leisure and the role of consumption through mHealth, particularly through processes of what Whitson (2013) describes as 'gamification'. Recognising the processes of gaming with many of the mHealth technologies, emerging work is beginning to explore this conflation between 'work and play' (Till, 2014) and the extent to which 'corporations have successfully convinced users that it is leisure, not labour' (Till, 2014, p. 449), despite the monetisation of data.

This blurring distinction between medical data and the commercialisation of health and wellness also raises a number of questions which sociologists can help answer. For example, sociology can shed light on questions of data ownership, revealing where points of exploitation occur, and where sites of resistance are apparent. Alternatively, a sociology of the new configurations of health care can more effectively outline the changing responsibilities of healthcare providers and their capacity to enable or discourage certain behaviours use that operate around mHealth applications. Increasingly, as health and wellness are commodified through mHealth, social theory and empirical work can reveal the role of particular groups, individuals and communities in resisting such process, or where they are complicit in supporting the system.

A key consideration in each of these areas is how users retain ownership and control of their data, which is a challenge that governments have yet to come to terms with, as it extends far beyond simple keeping of medical records. From the first round of the NHS Health App Library recommendations in 2013, research indicates that there were considerable gaps in the security features of data within these environments (Huckvale, Prieto, Tilney, Benghozi, & Car, 2015). Furthermore, it is alarming that increased commercialization of health data generates more privatised solutions to health care, new health data monopolies, and less capacity for users to move freely between providers. In response, there is a need for healthcare providers to restrict such trends or, at the very least, address the possibility of developing a universal data export format for personal health data. This is no minor proposal, especially given the expansion of mHealth applications beyond conventional health environments – such as Spotify mood choices. However, it is an urgent imperative since there will be nearly no utility in the NHS defining approved mHealth apps – or any such list – if all of the health data are locked into applications which are not on this list, or which do not identify themselves as mHealth environments. Indeed, the world's largest companies work more towards occupying space within the world's largest social media platforms, rather than consider building their own. As such, in order for mHealth to work, it is necessary for those who govern health care to work with these large mobile application developers, which means entering into a struggle over the ownership and exploitation of the data accrued through such platforms.

Mhealth, data distribution, and theories of surveillance

As a result of the data captured in digital self-tracking, the body becomes knowable to a range of institutions and organisation. To this end, a further trajectory of research must explore how mHealth technologies are being used by specific organisations to monitor others. This work is clearly derived from but could also inform theories of surveillance. In part, this is because communal self-tracking forms the basis of the next steps in mHealth and risk prevention, where individuals are encouraged to share data online with other self-trackers – albeit within proprietary databanks. Indeed, looking to the future, many of these trends are finding their way more formally into corporations, organisations and the pedagogic practices of different institutions. For example, in schools, there is growing support for the use of 'digital devices and software that allow students to collect, track, manipulate and share health-related data' (Gard, 2014, p. 838) particularly within Health and Physical Education (HPE) (see Cummiskey, 2011). In his paper on what he describes as the rise of eHPE, Gard (2014) fuses physical education's focus on public health discourses with developments in digital technology. Elsewhere, Williamson (2015) argues that young people's self-tracking through mobile devices should be seen as another dimension of governance within Physical Education. This approach reflects a broader trend in which schools are integrating data tracking and analytic technologies to monitor and measure student behaviours, a process described as the emergence of 'smart schools' (Williamson, 2014) or 'sentient schools' (Lupton, 2014b).

Elsewhere, a number of authors are pointing to the corporate use of technology to monitor the productivity and efficiency levels of their workers. For example, Gilmore (2015, p. 3) explores the 'complex ways wearable fitness technologies are transforming the concept of fitness at individual and institutional levels'. Till (2014, p. 452) reveals how fitness technologies are being integrated as employee wellness programs, suggesting that 'the data produced by devices, such as Fitbit, are conducive to existing techniques of corporate management in which workers are managed in terms of their quantified measures of productivity'. Individuals are being encouraged to use these technologies by insurance and medical organisations, as a way of tracking their lifestyles/health activities. In this sense, critical studies of mHealth provide an opportunity to explore the nuances of health surveillance.

Commenting in a special issue on 'Health' surveillance: new modes of monitoring bodies, populations, and polities', French and Smith (2013, p. 384) argue for greater critical attention on "health' surveillance, on its means and sometimes divergent ends'. Thus, where health data circulate within health assemblages, we need a better understanding of how it moves across different institutions. Critical mHealth studies are beginning to offer some insight. For example, Till (2014) suggests that the way in which health and commercial data are now used together reflects a 'syndromic surveillance' (Henning, 2004). Elsewhere, when examining the gap between the contexts for and practices with data, Fiore-Gartland and Neff (2015, p. 1467) focus on the 'social valences of data'. They identify six data valences (self-evidence, actionability, connection, transparency, 'truthiness' and discovery) and explore how these become mediated and are distinct across different social domains. Similarly, Lupton (2014b) provides important insights into the various modes of personal data production – private, pushed (encouraged), communal, imposed or exploited. Future research could begin to explore these modes of production within different social sites. Lupton (2014b) argues that 'pushed self-tracking departs from the private self-tracking mode in that the initial incentive for engaging in self-tracking comes from another actor or agency'.

We have yet fully to understand the impact of mHealth technologies on relationships which have, in recent years, been the focus of analysis of medical cyberspace and ehealth (Miah & Rich, 2008): doctor and patient, technology and bodies, patient and consumer. Furthermore, research is needed to explore the social impact of commercial child-tracking devices and applications, which allow parents to generate knowledge about their child's health, such as their physical activity (Williamson, 2015; Rich, in press), but it is likely that such devices could influence family relationships. Studies of this kind could for instance focus on the negotiation between different sites and value sets, such as the 'negotiation between commercial and community interests' (Barta & Neff, 2016). For Fiore-Gartland and Neff (2015, p. 1469) 'the renegotiation of these definitions occurs at the intersection of social domains and highlights the specific kinds of communication and mediation work that must be done around such data'. Such research agendas would (re)position mHealth 'ideologies and discourses that mobilise them beyond their transitory, ephemeral intervention in the lived environment' (Jethani, 2015, p. 40). Future research must also attend to the ways in which novel digital environments and different gatekeeping systems categorise and guide users towards particular mHealth technologies and not others.

Relatedly, it is useful to note that the taxonomy of health-related aspects of mHealth experiences is porous. Thus, separating out specific interests and biomedical markers that are addressed through specific apps has become increasingly difficult, because of the complexity of defining health. Specifying these boundaries will become harder over time, as an interest in well-being is present within the underlying principles of social media and the sharing economy. For instance, through image recognition software, Google is working on technology that can read the food content depicted within an image and make an assessment of its calorific content (Parkinson, 2015). Again, one can easily imagine how such data could be utilised – or sold to – organisations that have an interest in understanding the eating habits of a population, and yet one would not typically think of photo-sharing platforms like Instagram or Snapchat mHealth applications.

In this regard, mHealth is part of a complex assemblage of institutions, bodies, and discourses through which differing meanings of health become constituted and sometimes resisted. In this vein, we argue that there is an absence of insight into how different social groups negotiate and incorporate mhealth into everyday lives and of how moments of resistance to neoliberal systems of governance emerge. Certainly, some work has begun to explore such dimensions. For example, Barta and Neff (2016, p. 528) identify the quantified self-movement as a site for 'soft resistance' to big data practices 'allowing the community to be aligned with commercial purposes at times and to the individual control and autonomy over data at others'. Novel digital tools for sociological research enable researchers to understand conversations within mHealth communities, using approaches such as social network analysis or discourse analysis. For example, Jethani (2015, p. 39) argues that there is 'creative and political energy within practices of self-tracking' within the 'latencies' of the technological production of self-knowledge, for example, the possibility of self-tracking communities forming coalitions with other crowdfunding communities or open source developers.

Social inequalities, the production of knowledge and mHealth policies

Concerns about these systems are not just pertinent to individual interests; there are critical concerns about the way in which app data are distributed within proprietary systems, which can have an impact on how healthcare provision takes place. Concerns about data ownership and exploitation are emerging as one of the most important issues facing the healthcare industry today, since an ability to harness data will dictate the limits of solutions in the future. For now, the direction of travel is to lock up increasing amounts of our health-related data into proprietary systems, which limits the public utility they could generate, were such data actually publicly available. Below, we identify three key areas of ongoing and future research in relation to emerging questions about the social inequalities of mHealth.

First, we need to understand the capacity for governmentalities (Rose, 2000) through which the collation of big data on particular groups/populations may come to have significant implications. This connects with some of the enduring questions of social control within and through medicine, which have long occupied the work of sociologists of health and illness (Zola, 1972). Relatedly, there are questions about social inequities that arise in relation to how such data are utilised in the development of particular health promotion programs, interventions, or funding plans. For example, where algorithms and monitoring systems identify relationships between behaviours and particular individuals and groups, there may be occasions where such data are used to stigmatise the lifestyle of certain social groups. Also, theories of governmentality (as biopolitics) could examine how mHealth is utilised to identify how particular populations are deviating from the norm and how such data insights influence health policies, programs and targeted interventions.

Second, it is also necessary to ask how these data are being used as 'expert knowledge' which produces new risks associated with particular populations. The production of knowledge about and on people's bodies through quantified norms can be considered to be part of a 'biopolitics' of populations (Foucault, 1990) through which particular subjects are normalised and moralised. For example, in 2013, a report by think-tank Demos gathered media attention in the UK after it advised that 'people who lead healthy lifestyles should be rewarded with easier access to healthcare' (NHS, 2013). The report 'explores the impact of having a more 'responsible' population, and is largely focused on public health' (NHS, 2013). It gives some indication of the potential for such data to exclude those who do not conform to or who are unable to meet the expectations of health imperatives.

Third, whilst mHealth is celebrated for its ubiquitous potential, it is necessary also to be vigilant of the populations that are still absent from these environments and the inequalities and disparities this might exacerbate, as mHealth increasingly becomes a driver of health care. Insights from Livingstone and Helsper (2007) are instructive here, where they describe as 'a continuum of digital inclusion', particularly where access to mobile health is in its development. Empirical studies are needed to explore how different geographical, familial socio-economic, spatial, and cultural factors shape, limit or provide opportunity for the use of mHealth technologies. The neoliberal orientation of many mHealth technologies overlooks the complexity of health and the interrelationships that become constitutive of health and within which health practices and choices are made possible (Mol, 2008). The increasing use of global positioning systems (GPS) in apps and wearable technologies speaks both to the spatialities of mHealth and to the longstanding debates about the relationship between online and offline contexts.

Whilst there is evidence that populations are much more inclined to use technology to monitor their health, rather less attention has been paid to understanding how different geographical, familial socio-economic, spatial, and cultural factors shape, limit or provide opportunity for particular kinds of use of mHealth technologies and digital practices. The developments in GPS, gamification and wearable technologies demand conceptual approaches that avoid sharp demarcations between seemingly online/digital and offline/physical worlds and moves towards a non-dualist understanding of digital health practices. This compels us instead to think critically about spatiality and decisions about when, where, how and why we reach mHealth in our everyday practices. Multi-source data collection, spatial-time maps and other novel methods may become increasingly important in understanding complex everyday digital health practices in *real time*, space and place. Critical perspectives of this kind can help identify nuanced inequalities and disparities of mHealth across different sociocultural groups, shedding light on variations in mHealth literacy (Meppelink, van Weert, Haven, & Smit, 2015).

Conclusion: understanding the long tail of commercial mhealth

The sociology of health has begun to develop a critical reading of emerging mHealth technologies. Throughout this paper, we have explored these insights whilst also signalling theoretical directions for future research. The range of theoretical perspectives explored reveals that there is no single, comprehensive view of the body and mHealth, and each approach provokes different questions of materiality, representation and identity. Whilst we have focused on studies of consumer mHealth technologies oriented towards lifestyle and targeted at the individual, it is important to note that these technologies are increasingly being used within organizations and institutions for the purposes of monitoring others. In some ways, this has signalled a collapse of the ostensible boundaries between therapeutic medical technologies (treating medical conditions), and commercial mHealth technologies focused on the pursuit of self-enhancement. Indeed, this neat separation quickly disappears when we consider, for example, a GP referring patients to lifestyle-based apps to monitor their physical activity patterns.

It is tempting to encourage future research to focus solely on the established mobile media culture that is flourishing around health care today. However, present-day mobile devices must be seen as intermediary mechanisms, which are mostly ill equipped to deliver the efficiencies sought by its advocates. The next stage in the evolution of migratory data patterns is in the rise of wearable health technologies (wHealth) and their being enabled by the growth of the internet of things and a wider participatory culture of invention and discovery. Notwithstanding the capacity of the largest digital media organisations to acquire most of the outstanding propositions from new, start-up mHealth companies, one of the key consequences of this could be the not only further fragmentation of health data, but also its exponential growth in volume.

In 2004, Anderson conceived the notion of the 'long tail' (2004), which describes the new economy of digital culture, where the larger volume of low users exceeds the influence of the high peak of fewer users. In a similar vein, one may talk about the long tail of health-care reform being dependent on the optimisation and exploitation of data. Such trends signal a need to consider the connections between digital technologies and broader biomedical spheres. Yet, for all of the discourse around the need for open data initiatives, the mHealth industry is progressively undermining this prospect year after year, leaving healthcare providers and governors increasingly less able to meet the demands on their system. We have explored the underpinning trajectory of such trends, considering how new forms of self-tracking technology are situated within wider technological processes. The rise of the internet of things, the growth of citizen science, new implant technology and the emergence of DIY gene editing kits are examples of trends within this field, and each deserves greater scrutiny from digital sociologists. Together, these artefacts within our technological culture reveal a future of self-tracking in health care that is increasingly automated and increasingly invasive, the utilisation of which may eventually undermine the ethics of healthcare provision. At the very least, it will ensure greater economic and political power for those organisations which store personal health data.

On this understanding, there are many other aspects of mHealth that require further consideration as one looks towards the early stages of these future trends. The speed at which technologies are developing raises questions about the adequacy of theoretical frameworks and method. For example, Jethani (2015, p. 36) asserts that the emergence of wearable technologies and biosensors has focused attention on 'how sensors are being projected inwards into the body' in ways that 'reorients the study of self-tracking practices as new media'. Ultimately, the end point of digital health solutions may be a complete erosion of autonomy in a world where this control is assumed by intelligent machines, capable of providing the appropriate response to undesirable fluctuations in our health status. Whether or not we would be better off as a population for handing over such control to autonomous systems remains to be seen, but it is crucial to recognise that such a system would be underpinned by a very different set of assumptions about what constitutes autonomy or free will. At the very least, wHealth describes a completely novel set of interfaces between the user and the self-tracking technology, which characterises a new field of investigation into how technology is changing health care.

Disclosure statement

No potential conflict of interest was reported by the authors.

References

Alrige, M., & Chatterjee, S. (2015). Toward a taxonomy of wearable technologies in healthcare. In B. Donnellan et al. (Eds.), *New horizons in design science: Broadening the research agenda, volume 9073 of the series lecture notes in computer science* (pp. 496–504). Cham: Springer International Publishing.

Anderson, C. (2004). The long tail, *Wired*. Retrieved from http://www.wired.com/2004/10/tail/

Andrejevic, M. (2005). The work of watching one another: Lateral surveillance, risk, and governance. *Surveillance & Society*, 2(4), 479–497.

Andrejevic, M., & Burdon, M. (2015). Defining the sensor society. *Television & New Media*, 16(1), 19–36. doi:10.1177/1527476414541552

Barta, K., & Neff, G. (2016). Technologies for sharing: Lessons from quantified self about the political economy of platforms. *Information, Communication & Society*, 19(4), 518–531. doi:10.1080/1369118X.2015.1118520

Bauman, Z. (2007). *Consuming life*. Cambridge, UK: Polity.

Boxall, A. (2014). *2014 is the year of health and fitness apps, says Google*. Retrieved December 11, 2014, from http://www.digitaltrends.com/mobile/google-play-store-2014-most-downloaded-apps/

Cummiskey, M. (2011). There's an app for that: Smartphone use in health and physical education. *The Journal of Physical Education, Recreation & Dance*, 82(8), 24–30. doi:10.1080/07303084.2011.10598672

Deleuze, G. (1988). *Spinoza: Practical philosophy*. San Francisco, CA: City Light.

European Commission. (2010). *A digital agenda for Europe: Communication from the commission*. Brussels: European Commission.

Fiore-Gartland, B., & Neff, G. (2015). Communication, mediation, and the expectations of data: Data valences across health and wellness communities. *International Journal of Communication*, 9, 1466–1484. ISSN 1932-803.

Foucault, M. (1988). Technologies of the self. In L. Martin, H. Gutman, & P. Hutton (Eds.), *Technologies of the self: A seminar with Michel Foucault* (pp. 16–49). Amherst: The University of Massachusetts Press.

Foucault, M. (1990). *The history of sexuality: An introduction, volume I. Translated by Robert Hurley*. New York, NY: Vintage Books.

Fox, N. J. (2011). The ill-health assemblage: Beyond the body-with-organs. *Health Sociology Review*, 20(4), 359–371. doi:10.5172/hesr.2011.20.4.359

Fox, N. J. (2016). Health sociology from post-structuralism to the new materialisms. *Health*, 20(1), 62–74.

Fox, S., & Duggan, M. (2013). *Tracking for health*. Retrieved from http://www.pewinternet.org/2013/01/28/tracking-for-health/

French, M., & Smith, G. (2013). 'Health' surveillance: New modes of monitoring bodies, populations, and polities. *Critical Public Health*, 23(4), 383–392. doi:10.1080/09581596.2013.838210

Fries, C. J. (2008). Governing the health of the hybrid self: Integrative medicine, neoliberalism, and the shifting biopolitics of subjectivity. *Health Sociology Review*, 17(4), 353–367. doi:10.5172/hesr.451.17.4.353

Galloway, A. (2004). Intimations of everyday life: Ubiquitous computing and the city. *Cultural Studies*, 18(2–3), 324–408.

Gard, M. (2014). eHPE: A history of the future. *Sport, Education and Society*, 19(6), 827–845. doi:10.1080/13573322.2014.938036

Gilmore, J. N. (2015). Everywear: The quantified self and wearable fitness technologies. *New Media and Society*, 1–16. doi:10.1177/1461444815588768

Haggerty, K. D., & Ericson, R. V. (2000). The surveillant assemblage. *British Journal of Sociology*, 5(51), 605–622. doi:10.1080/00071310020015280

Henderson, S., & Petersen, A. (Eds.). (2002). *Consuming health: The commodification of health care*. Routledge: London.

Henning, K. J. (2004). Overview of syndromic surveillance: What is syndromic surveillance? *MMWR*, 53(Suppl), 5–11.

Huckvale, K., Prieto, J. T., Tilney, M., Benghozi, P-J., & Car, J. (2015). Unaddressed privacy risks in accredited health and wellness apps: A cross-sectional systematic assessment. *BMC Medicine*, 13(1), 214. doi: 10.1186/s12916-015-0444-y

Jethani, S. (2015). Mediating the body: Technology, politics and epistemologies of self. *Communication, Politics and Culture*, 47(3), 34–43.

Livingstone, S., & Helsper, E. (2007). Gradations in digital inclusion: Children, young people and the digital divide. *New Media and Society*, 9(4), 671–696. doi:10.1177/1461444807080335

Lupton, D. (2012). M-health and health promotion: The digital cyborg and surveillance society. *Social Theory and Health*, 10, 229–244. doi:10.1057/sth.2012.6

Lupton, D. (2013a). The digitally engaged patient: Self-monitoring and self-care in the digital health Era. *Social Theory and Health*, 11(3), 256–270.

Lupton, D. (2013b). Understanding the human machine. *IEEE Technology and Society Magazine*, 32(4), 25–30. doi:10.1109/MTS.2013.2286431

Lupton, D. (2014a). Beyond techno-utopia: Critical approaches to digital health technologies. *Societies*, 4, 706–711. doi:10.3390/soc4040706

Lupton, D. (2014b, August 27). Self-tracking modes: Reflexive self-monitoring and data practices. Paper presented at the 'Imminent Citizenships: Personhood and Identity Politics in the Informatic Age' workshop, ANU, Canberra.

Mayer-Schönberger, V., & Cukier, K. (2013). *Big data: A revolution that will transform how we live, work, and think*. New York, NY: Houghton Mifflin Harcourt.

Meppelink, C. S., van Weert, J. C. M., Haven, C. J., & Smit, E. G. (2015). The effectiveness of health animations in audiences with different health literacy levels: An experimental study. *Journal of Medical Internet Research, 17*(1), e11. doi:10.2196/jmir.3979

Miah, A., & Rich, E. (2008). *The medicalization of cyberspace.* Oxon: Routledge.

Millington, B. (2015). 'Quantify the invisible': Notes toward a future of posture. *Critical Public Health,* doi:10.1080/09581596.2015.1085960

Mol, A. (2008). *The logic of care: Health and the problem of patient choice.* London: Routledge.

NHS. (2013). *'Reward people who 'live healthily' says think-tank'.* Retrieved from http://www.nhs.uk/news/2013/03March/Pages/Reward-people-who-live-healthily-says-think-tank.aspx

NHS England. (2014). *Five year forward view.* Retrieved February 24, 2015, from https://www.england.nhs.uk/wp-content/uploads/2014/10/5yfv-web.pdf

Parkinson, H. J. (2015, June 2). Google wants to count the calories in your Instagram food porn, *The Guardian,* Retrieved July 11, 2015, from http://www.theguardian.com/technology/2015/jun/02/google-calories-instagram-food-porn

Powell, A. C., Landman, A. B., & Bates, D. W. (2014). In search of a few good apps. *Journal of The American Medical Association, 311*(18), 1851–1852. doi:10.1001/jama.2014.2564

Proteus. (2015, September 10). *U.S. FDA accepts first digital medicine new drug application for Otsuka and Proteus digital health – proteus digital health.* (n.d.). Retrieved February 25, 2016, from http://www.proteus.com/press-releases/u-s-fda-accepts-first-digital-medicine-new-drug-application-for-otsuka-and-proteus-digital-health/

Research2Guidance. (2014). *mHealth App Developer Economics 2014 The State of the Art of mHealth App Publishing.* Retrieved from: http://research2guidance.com/r2g/research2guidance-mHealth-App-Developer-Economics-2014.pdf

Rich, E., & Miah, A. (2014). Understanding digital health as public pedagogy: A critical framework. *Societies, 4,* 296–315. doi:10.3390/soc4020296

Rich, E. (in press). Childhood, surveillance and mHealth technologies: The surveillance of children's bodies. In E. Taylor & T. Rooney (Eds.), *Surveillance futures: Social and ethical implications of new technologies for children and young people.* London: Ashgate.

Rose, N. (2000). Government and control. *British Journal of Criminology, 40*(2), 321–339. doi:10.1093/bjc/40.2.321

Ruckenstein, M. (2014). Visualized and interacted life: Personal analytics and engagements with data doubles. *Societies, 4,* 68–84. doi:10.3390/soc4010068

Swan, M. (2012). Health 2050: The realization of personalized medicine through crowdsourcing, the quantified self, and the participatory Biocitizen. *Journal of Personalized Medicine, 2*(4), 93–118. doi:10.3390/jpm2030093

Till, C. (2014). Exercise as labour: Quantified self and the transformation of exercise into labour. *Societies, 4,* 446–462. doi:10.3390/soc4030446

Whitson, J. (2013). Gaming the quantified self. *Surveillance and. Society, 11*(1/2), 163–176.

Williamson, B. (2014). Governing software: Networks, databases and algorithmic power in the digital governance of education. *Learning, Media & Technology,* doi:10.1080/17439884.2014.924527

Williamson, B. (2015). Algorithmic skin: Health-tracking technologies, personal analytics and the biopedagogies of digitized health and physical education. *Sport, Education and Society, 20*(1), 133–151. doi:10.1080/13573322.2014.962494

World Health Organization. (2011). *Mhealth: New horizons for health through mobile technologies: Based on the findings of the second global survey on eHealth* (Global Observatory for eHealth Series, Volume 3). Geneva: WHO Press.

Zola, I. (1972). Medicine as an institution of social control. *Sociological Review, 20*(4), 487–504. doi:10.1111/j.1467-954X.1972.tb00220.x

Are we fit yet? English adolescent girls' experiences of health and fitness apps

Annaleise Depper and P. David Howe

ABSTRACT

In recent years, society has witnessed a proliferation of digital technologies facilitate new ways to monitor young people's health. This paper explores a group of English adolescent girls' understandings of 'health' promoted by health and fitness related technologies. Five focus group meetings with the same 8 girls, aged between 14 and 17, were conducted to explore their experiences of using health and fitness apps. The girls' understandings of the digitised body are examined through a Foucauldian lens, with particular attention to conceptualisations of bio-power and technologies of the self. The data reveal how the girls negotiated, and at times critiqued, the multiple health discourses that are manifest through digital health technologies and performative health culture. The results emphasise that individual-based applications (apps) remove the social and interactive elements of physical activity valued by the girls. This research highlights the possibilities digital technologies provide for health promotion, yet also illuminates the limitations of these technologies if used uncritically and inappropriately.

Introduction

In this paper, we examine the views of a group of Sports Leaders, within an English state grammar school for girls, around engaging with health and fitness related apps and wearable technologies. We investigate the socio-cultural implications of utilising these devices upon their embodied health and their broader understanding of what it means to be 'healthy'. Our research illustrates how a group of adolescent girls valued the social possibilities of engaging in physical activity, whilst criticised digital technologies for removing the interactive elements of traditional sport and for promoting narrow health ideals.

In recent years, digital technologies related to health and fitness promotion have been emphasised as a technical solution to adolescents' sedentary lifestyles (Sport England, 2015). Due to the ubiquity of interactive technologies within adolescents' lives, 'apps' (specialised programs downloadable to mobile devices) have particularly resonated with young individuals (Ofcom, 2011). Over the past decade, the numerous readily available health and fitness technologies have arguably served a Western agenda to combat the so-called 'obesity epidemic' (Rich & Miah, 2014), which has been the subject of academic dispute over its exaggeration and uncertainty (see Rich, 2011a). Indeed, digital devices contradict with government policy rhetoric that strives for a broader approach to reducing health disparities, as opposed to 'focusing on individuals' specific health-related behaviours' (Lupton, 2015, p. 176).

In schools, digital health technologies have begun to be employed to promote physical activity amongst young people (Millington, 2009). Apps and wearable technologies function as pedagogical devices, facilitating an interactive space through which young people can learn how to value a desirable body in the pursuit of functional health (Rich & Miah, 2014). As adolescents are encouraged to monitor and regulate their bodies, digital health technologies are arguably intrusive methods within the existing performative spaces of schools to serve wider societal health intervention. According to Evans, Rich, and Holroyd (2004), these body performance and perfection codes unjustly place 'moral obligation and blame on individuals for their health/problems' (p. 139). This neoliberal, 'ideology of healthism' pervades the lives of adolescents beyond schooling, as digital health technologies expand the parameters of surveillance upon the young body.

This paper begins with a review of academic literature that examines digital health technologies through notions of embodiment and subjectivity. At the forefront of this paper is this concept of embodiment and specific attention is given to how these notions inform our understanding of the embodied identities of both the participants and the focus group facilitator. We then explore Foucault's conceptualisation of bio-power in relation to understandings of the digitised, 'healthy' body. Subsequently, we examine digital health within popular pedagogical spaces, as they extend the boundaries through which adolescents can engage in self-monitoring to conform to culturally and socially acceptable body 'ideals'.

Situating embodied subjectivities

With the growing commodification and privatisation of digital health technologies, health and fitness apps have the potential for 'even more intense forms of surveillance, normalisation and potential "Othering" of students whose data do not conform to set expectations' (Lupton, 2015, p. 128). It is important to consider the implications of these restrictive health discourses upon adolescents' embodied practices, subjectivities and discursive understandings of health. As McEvilly, Atencio, Verheul, and Jess (2013) emphasise, health discourses significantly influence 'children's sense of self, which is directly linked with being physical and embodied' (p. 733).

Specifically, this research engages with the ways in which a group of female Sports Leaders subjectively negotiated the multiple discourses of 'health' within digital health technologies. Girls at this English grammar school were awarded the status of Sports Leaders by the Head of the Physical Education (PE) Department for taking on various responsibilities at the school, such as assisting at sports related school events, being the captain of a sports team, umpiring sports fixtures and being positive sporting role models to other girls. We are reflexive that the embodiment of both the participants and the focus group facilitator was inextricably linked to the data collection process; this particular group of white, middle-class girls had an embodied sense of self as 'sporty' individuals, while the girls subjectively interpreted and related to the facilitator's body as young, white and also 'sporty'. For example, the girls collectively referred to individuals who might be considered as inactive or 'obese' as distinctly 'other' to those present in the focus group. We have embraced this importance of acknowledging the self as part of the subjectivities within the data collection, analysis and research writing at 'every stage of the research' (Guillemin & Gillam, 2004, p. 274).

Foucault and the discursive construction of the digitised 'healthy' body

The work of Foucault around discourse, bio-power and normalisation has received extensive attention across digital and health sociology. Digital health technologies have intensified the imperative to be healthy within modern society, which Foucault (1984) critiques, is 'the duty of each and objective for all' (p. 277). Normalisation as a form of bio-power remains prevalent to understanding rising concerns over the so-called 'obesity epidemic' and has given rise to moral imperatives to be healthy, virtuous bio-citizens (Harwood, 2009). According to Foucault (1978), through 'continuous regulatory and corrective mechanisms' (p. 144) within society, monitoring is used to normalise individuals into docile bodies. Foucault refers to Jeremy Bentham's 'plan for the panopticon as the paradigm of a disciplinary technology' in order to bring together disciplinary power and knowledge (Rabinow, 1991, p. 18), the joining of which Foucault refers to as 'technologies' that 'come together around the objectification of the body' (Rabinow, 1991, p. 17). The strength of this panoptic arrangement and disciplinary power emerges from normalising judgement and plays a fundamental role in normalising and correcting 'anomalies' of the overweight or obese body.

A wealth of literature has applied Foucault's concept of bio-power to emphasise that the adolescent body is particularly vulnerable to dominant discourses around the apparent 'obesity epidemic' (Gard & Wright, 2001; Rich, 2011b). Rich (2011b), for example, critically examines the bio-pedagogical strategies of new health imperatives that are ubiquitous in 'both the formal and popular pedagogic sites of learning about the health and body' (p. 66) and facilitate the means for young people to self-monitor. This Foucauldian lens is central to our own interpretation of the participants' experiences of digital health within this study.

Digital health and popular pedagogical spaces

The work of Foucault has been influential in guiding a critical examination of digital health and self-tracking. However, much of academic research around self-tracking technologies has uncritically engaged with these devices as instrumental tools for children's health intervention, particularly within the context of schooling (Nichols, Davis, McCord, Schmidt, & Slezak, 2009; Quraishi & Quraishi, 2012). For example, Cummiskey (2011) highlights the functional integration of technology within the PE curriculum, such as the MapMyRun˙ app, which allows pupils to calculate and monitor their physical activity levels. Research has also explored the functional use of bodily measurement devices (Nichols et al., 2009) and video games as a form of exercise and track body movement (known as exergaming; Vander Schee & Boyles, 2010), yet studies rarely critically engage with the ethical implications of these technologies on children's long-term well-being.

Increasingly, research from a more critical perspective has examined the popular cultural spaces through which adolescents interact and learn about their own bodies and health outside of education (Millington, 2009; Rich, 2011a). These studies critically engage with the frequently restrictive health discourses inherent in adolescents' everyday informal spaces that entice individuals to surveil their own bodies. For example, weight loss reality television shows, such as The Biggest Loser®, include bio-pedagogical strategies to prompt individuals to 'undertake surveillance of their own and others' bodies' (Rich, 2011a, p. 3). Such strategies have extended to more interactive, exergaming technologies. For example, the Nintendo Wii Fit® has been critiqued for encouraging children to reflect on their own body in comparison to the norm 'as they undertake their journey towards self-governance and thus "a better you"' (Ohman, Almqvist, Meckbach, & Quennerstedt, 2014, p. 202). Wearable health monitoring devices, such as the Nike+ FuelBand® and Fitbit®, have further transformed the temporal space through which individuals' body data is monitored. Rich and Miah (2009) emphasise how weight monitoring technologies facilitate 'prosthetic surveillance' and have renegotiated the corporeal boundaries of individuals' virtual and real bodies. Despite a growing critical analysis of digital health, much of this research engages with artefacts within popular media and consumer culture, and the voices of young individuals interacting with these digital spaces are often absent from these accounts.

Methodology and analysis

This research was approved by the university's ethics committee, which highlighted we had support from an English state grammar school for girls to hold 5 focus group meetings with 8 girls; three of the girls were aged 14 and the rest were aged 17. The Head of the PE department distributed a poster advert to Sports Leaders, inviting them to assist in a 'Research study – using fitness apps in PE'. We provided an information sheet for parents/guardians and a 'child-friendly' information sheet for pupils, clearly detailing the girls' roles in the focus groups, confidentiality of the data storage and their rights to withdraw from the research at any time. In the interest of ensuring anonymity, the names of the pupils, teachers and school have been replaced with pseudonyms. Over a 5-week period, the primary investigator met with the same girls for 40 minutes during their lunch break, once a week.

Prior to the focus groups, the primary investigator prepared a guide containing open-ended questions that allowed flexibility to adjust to the participants' experiences. Task-orientated activities enabled the girls to actively engage in health and fitness apps of their choosing, after which the researcher facilitated rich discussion of the girls' perspectives of the apps. In comparison to one-to-one interviews, the participant-led tasks facilitated opportunities for the girls to discuss and challenge dominant understandings of health and fitness technologies. Moreover, we are reflexive that the perceptions of the participants in this study are not representative of all adolescents and we maintain the belief that meeting with a smaller sample of the same girls over a period of time enhanced the richness of discussions than had we conducted focus groups with multiple groups of adolescents.

Our analysis centred on interpreting the adolescent girls' embodied understandings of health and fitness apps within the discursive context of societal health. Foucault's (1988) work resonates with our attention to the intertwining of discourse, knowledge and power through the girls' understandings of digital health technologies. While a Foucauldian discourse analysis is advantageous in examining language and 'the ways in which discourse constructs subjectivity, selfhood and power relations' (Sparkes & Smith, 2014, pp. 136–137), the focus of our analysis was to guide a more in-depth study of the ways in which the girls embodied and negotiated health discourses inherent in digital health technologies.

Specifically, we adapted Markula and Silk's (2011) poststructuralist approach for analysing interviews, to explore the patterns and themes emerging through the focus groups. After transcribing the focus group audio data, we firstly inductively searched for and identified themes relevant to our research question and purpose. We then followed an analysis of the themes through engaging with the intersections and discrepancies between the themes, in order to produce a concise list of three new themes. Finally, we made connections between these new themes and 'power relations, theory and previous literature' (Markula & Silk, 2011, p. 109). Our discussion of the data in the subsequent chapters is centred on these final three themes.

We mobilise various Foucauldian theoretical concepts to further support our analysis, particularly Foucault's concepts of bio-power and technologies of the self in order to analyse the participants' engagement in digital health technologies as pedagogical and discursive sites. This research departs from understanding health and fitness apps solely as 'technologies of dominance', in order to capture the repressive yet also creative opportunities, uncertainties and contradictions within digital health. Thus, we seek not the contingency of a discourse of 'health' as dominating marginal ones, but an exploration of the girls' negotiation of numerous discourses of health embedded in digital technologies.

The digital, self-tracking adolescent generation

Our analysis and discussion of the focus group data first turns to the ways in which the adolescent girls reinforced the societal acceptance that engaging in self-tracking technologies was a ubiquitous part of their digital generation. This was evident when the girls agreed with Jessica's assumption that health and fitness apps are a 'useful', accessible function to all young people:

Jessica: People our age are surrounded by the media and everyone's always on their phone, so [fitness] apps are something useful to have, because obviously you're always going to have your phone on you at this age.

This emphasised the girls' position as 'digital natives', able to incorporate technologies into their everyday lives. Although the girls did not reflect upon class issues, it is important to consider the girls' position as relatively privileged, middle-class individuals. Their assumption that all adolescents are surrounded by technology can perhaps be explained by their status as grammar school pupils; the girls rarely reflected upon individuals beyond their particular social worlds whose differing social, cultural and economic circumstances might limit their use of electronic devices.

Social media was a significant part of the participants' engagement in digital health technologies and this further emphasised the appeal of the interactive fitness devices amongst adolescents. During the focus groups, the girls perceived that individuals were likely to share their progress on health and fitness apps through social media for competitive and motivational reasons and that other individuals could be inspired by functional, healthy behaviour:

Sarah: It [Strava® running and cycling app] links with a lot of social media, so you can post your ride or run on Facebook®, so that could motivate other people to do it when they see that you've done it.

Charlotte: … so therefore there's an element of competition, so you want to try and beat each other.

This reinforced how health and fitness apps can facilitate significant social opportunities through online communities. Marwick's (2012) understanding of social surveillance as the interpersonal, 'positive, supportive social effects' (p. 391) of mutual sharing on social media is particularly relevant to the girls' discussion. However, the way in which individuals might potentially be exploited or subject to peer pressure through use of social media alongside fitness apps was absent from the girls' narratives.

Throughout the focus groups, the girls frequently reflected on how other individuals might respond to health and fitness apps, particularly those that were disengaged from sport and physical activity, whom they perceived needed increased motivation. This was highlighted in the following discussion:

Sarah: I know some people and they download them, they have folders with their apps in, like fitness apps, but they never use them they just have them.

Researcher: Why do you think they have them?

Jessica: Maybe they want to use them, but they don't really, they just like to look good … like 'I do sport, I am fit'.

The participants perceived that some girls would conform to techniques of self-monitoring and regulation through health and fitness related apps to give the impression of being a 'fit' individual to their peers. It is important to remember that this group of individuals were Sports Leaders who engaged in regular physical activity for enjoyment and thus, they were cynical of individuals who might pretend to use apps to fit into this 'sporty' ideal that was valued by the girls. The girls demonstrated a critical awareness that individuals might strive to appear to engage in self-discipline to gain the supportive effects of conforming to an 'ideal' body. This resonates with the discourses around the online trend of 'fitspiration', where individuals share fitness related content designed to 'inspire viewers towards a healthier lifestyle by promoting exercise and healthy food', in order to achieve positive body image (Tiggemann & Zaccardo, 2015, p. 61).

The girls emphasised that health and fitness apps illustrating the transformation of a body could significantly motivate other individuals to engage in fitness pursuits. This emerged when the girls were encouraged to consider the potential negative consequences of health and fitness apps. The following discussion emphasises how the girls perceived that some app users might be demotivated by solely viewing an athlete model demonstrate fitness workouts, while observing another individual gradually transform their body could be more motivating:

Millie: Maybe the body image it presents … like on a lot of apps, the people doing it looked like they were athletes already. And maybe they should have more people that look normal.

Jessica:	Yeah, they should have people that look more normal and then show their progression, instead of having really fit people with six packs already.
Emma:	Yeah, it might be a bit intimidating.
Millie:	They might think like 'I don't look like that' and then they don't use the app.
Grace:	Yeah, if they showed them at gradual stages it would probably be a lot more motivating that just seeing this perfect body that it has at the end.

This transformation discourse and the idea of viewing the 'before and after' image of an individuals' fitness progress frequently emerges across young people's popular and social media. Although the girls critiqued the lack of 'normal' bodies and preoccupation with the 'perfect body' on apps, they reinforced restrictive health discourses inherent in the gradual progression *towards* an 'ideal'. This highlights the pedagogical nature of individuals' engagement with digital technologies; through which adolescents can learn how to transform one's body to achieve the 'appropriate' body and become healthy bio-citizens (Wright & Halse, 2014). It is again important to emphasise that the girls were not entirely self-reflexive and often reflected upon the responses of other individuals, whom they thought lacked the motivation to engage in health and sporting pursuits.

In cases where the girls highlighted how they engaged with health and fitness apps, this was predominantly for the purposes of self-tracking and improving their fitness. According to the girls, running related apps such as MapMyRun®, facilitated this self-monitoring:

| Sarah: | I think it's just to give advice and track how you're doing, like I find that my running app is quite useful because you can remember what you've done so you can be like I missed one day but oh, I did that the other day so it's fine. You can look back at what you have done. |

The participants agreed that these types of apps were particularly motivating as they provided tangible proof of their efforts. This emphasised neoliberal discourses around the self-responsibility to track and monitor one's body in order to achieve culturally valued definitions of health (Harwood, 2009). These opportunities for prosthetic surveillance significantly reinforced a 'corporeal' responsibility upon the girls and facilitated new ways to monitor their bodies and fitness. Foucault's conceptualisation of technologies of the self is useful in understanding the girls' engagement with health and fitness apps. Markula (2004) emphasises that this concept signifies a shift from the disciplined individual to one that engages in 'practices of freedom [to] enable a creative transformation of the self' (p. 304). This notion is central to 'moving beyond simplistic notions of socialisation to a more complex understanding of how the operation of power works to connect the self with the social' (Wright, O'Flynn, & Macdonald, 2006, p. 708). Throughout the focus groups it was evident that, through deciding to engage in particular digital health technologies, the girls held the freedom to experience the managing of their bodies along particular social lines, conforming to the moral imperatives associated with being a healthy bio-citizen.

'Healthy' and self-responsible bio-citizens

During the focus groups, the girls emphasised that the characteristics defining a healthy individual were 'Happy – physically and mentally, balanced diet, active, outside, good night's sleep'. References to an illness-free or slender body as representative of health were notably absent. Discourses around the social, emotional and physical dimensions of healthy lifestyles elucidated the girls' hesitations to label a particular slender 'ideal' as healthy. The girls' understandings of health moved beyond the discourse of healthism that is frequently emphasised across the everyday practices of schooling (Halse, Honey, & Boughtwood, 2007) and also the informal spaces of digital health and popular media, whereby slender bodies are often representative of health and fitness.

When given the opportunity to engage in health and fitness apps during the focus groups, the girls criticised apps (such as Nike+ Training Club®) for reducing social interaction and emphasised that the individual nature of apps would be detrimental if implemented in their PE lessons:

Millie: I mean you could do the Nike (Nike+ Training Club®) app circuit in just the gym, you could just follow that, but then you can't really do other sports like Rounders, you can only use it for certain things.

Emma: I think apps are more for your independent use ... like in a PE lesson you can't really use it, there would be lack of human interaction and communication with your teacher.

Although the girls emphasised that this holistic social interaction was important within school, they perceived that health and fitness apps could be beneficial for helping individuals focus on improving their health outside of school. For example, the girls were uncritical about the way in which individuals should be accountable for their own health and agreed with Emma's perception that apps reinforced the message that:

Emma: ... individual people are responsible for their own health.

When considering the girls' compliance with dominant health imperatives, it is important to acknowledge the significance of their status as Sports Leaders within a relatively privileged grammar school. Previous research has emphasised that middle-class adolescents comply with dominant health discourses in the pursuit of moral behaviour and a functional body (Wachs & Chase, 2013). The girls' perspectives that other individuals are accountable for their own health arguably reinforced the girls' own presentation of the self as responsible bio-citizens. This neoliberal discourse around the social responsibility for monitoring one's individual health dominates contemporary understandings of health and weight. Drawing upon Foucault's (1988) conceptualisation that power and knowledge come together to normalise particular bodily ideals and practices; we can understand that the girls enforced the normalising judgement of health as an individual responsibility upon their own and other individuals' bodies. The power of these health and body discourses circulated through the multiple pedagogical spaces the participants engaged with in their everyday lives. While at times the girls emphasised holistic understandings of health, they also emphasised restrictive definitions of health. It is important to note here, as Lupton (1995) emphasises, that 'subjects are never fully governed by discourse nor fully capable of stepping outside discourse' (p. 137).

During the focus groups, discussions emerged around the girls' understandings of the so-called 'obesity epidemic'. When encouraged to consider how apps relate to the health of wider society, the girls reinforced dominant discourses around the importance of being healthy citizens to improve society. The girls perceived that growing levels of obesity are a problem in society and health and fitness apps could serve as a free, accessible method for overweight individuals to take responsibility for their own health. They all agreed this would reduce strain on the National Health Service:

> Emma: In the past few years obesity has become more of an issue, you hear about it a lot more, so I guess apps can make people more aware of size, motivate people more to do exercise because people who were just looking through their phone and see a free app they might try it out and find out they might actually enjoy it and do more exercise.

In particular, Emma emphasised that apps encourage individuals to be 'more aware of size', and therefore apps reinforced the visibility of this discourse around monitoring the body to lose weight. Foucault's (1988) concept of bio-power is relevant to understanding how health monitoring apps play a role in normalising and correcting 'deviances' such as obesity amongst individuals. Through disciplinary practices, individuals internalise 'the control mechanisms through the body discipline' and are thus governed by themselves; their own responsibility to 'obtain the healthy look' (Markula, 2001, p. 254). Through Foucault's (1988) notion of the panopticon, we can understand how the participants were subjected to wider societal regimes of the dominant discourse of 'healthy' weight norms and moral panic surrounding the 'obesity epidemic'. Localised in the participants' bodies, the girls emphasised the individual imperative to direct surveillance upon one's own health, such as through engaging with digital technologies, in order to reduce the costs of obesity on the welfare state.

Although the girls conformed to dominant obesity discourses, they were nevertheless critical of the business of app-making to make money on individuals trying to lose weight. When encouraged to consider why apps were made, the girls all agreed with Emma's perception that health and fitness monitoring apps could be perceived as appealing business investments:

> Emma: … it's a popular idea with people because quite a lot of people will want to get fit or lose weight maybe because just society and the media and stuff like that, so I guess it is quite a good way to make money.

This narrative emphasised the commercial marketing of self-monitoring technologies to capitalise on attempts to achieve the healthy bio-citizen 'ideal'. Jutel (2006) posits that the 'disease of "overweight" is a perfect and fertile ground for commercial exploitation' (p. 2275). Moreover, societal beliefs around the 'ideal' body 'underpin a multi-billion dollar diet, gym, self-help, television and pharmaceutical approach to weight maintenance' (Jutel, 2006, p. 2275). Although the health of today's youth has been argued to be a significant target for this neoliberal exploitation and intervention (Lupton, 2013), this group of female adolescents were critically aware of the commercial business ventures of apps.

The girls' critique: apps promote 'ideal' bodies and remove social interaction

Throughout the focus group meetings, the participants demonstrated a critical under-standing that apps frequently promote slender body shapes as representative of an 'ideal'. The girls perceived that the female bodies presented on the apps, such as Popsugar Active® (an app that allows users to create custom routines and share workouts with friends), were unrealistic and likely to result in demotivating other girls. For example, Zoe suggested:

> Zoe: It could put people off if they see these people with perfect bodies that have done it, they'll think that I'm obviously not good enough to do this, maybe, I should do something else different, a bit less intimidating, but then other people would find it quite inspirational, thinking 'oh if I keep going with this then I'll be able to do this'.

The girls were further critical that the models in the apps had often undergone cosmetic surgery or edited their images in order to appear as 'perfect', which they critiqued was impossible to achieve. This group of girls demonstrated the agency to consider how narrow representations of the toned, slender body promoted by the health and fitness apps could be demotivating for some yet function as enabling processes for others. Foucault's (1988) concept of technologies of the self helps us understand the creative reconstruction of the body through practices of freedom that help to monitor and transform one's bodies in line with the social norm. This is significant when considering how the adolescent girls had the freedom to either resist or comply with health imperatives. According to Wright et al. (2006), these differing responses can occur 'even in cases where they [young people] are aware of social critiques of the work of the media and other agencies in promoting body ideals that are unattainable by most' (p. 708). The girls were conscious and at times critical that, through health and fitness apps, individuals are encouraged to engage in self-monitoring and regulation; or as Foucault (1988) articulates, 'a certain number of operations on their own bodies and souls' (p. 15) in the pursuit of a bio-citizen ideal.

The girls were particularly critical of health and fitness apps that used the term 'BMI' (body mass index) to classify individuals as having either a 'normal' or 'abnormal' weight. This emerged during a discussion of the Wii Fit® game's promotion of 'ideal' weight as having stigmatising effects upon individuals:

> Emma: ... because my sister's really muscly, she's considered a bit overweight, even though she's absolutely not, but because of the weight on the thing, it says your overweight, but you're not.
> Millie: Yeah.
> Emma: So yeah I guess that could be quite negative.
> Millie: It's not very accurate.
> Emma: Exactly, it can't look at you and see what you actually look like.

Both girls emphasised that BMI measuring was a generalisable and inaccurate approach for those with additional muscle mass and it was necessary to subjectively evaluate an individual's health. Through Foucault's concepts of self-governance and bio-power, we can understand how exergames, such as the Wii Fit®, can become problematic as they assert pressure upon young individuals to regulate their bodies according to normative standards and socially acceptable BMI levels (Ohman et al., 2014). While at times young people might seemingly reinforce dominant discourses of health, Beausoleil (2009) emphasises that 'young people's bodies are not completely regulated by the current socially prescribed health imperative' (p. 94). This resonates with the ways in which the girls' reinforcement of restrictive health discourses did not endure throughout every focus group discussion. We, therefore, depart from the view of adolescents as cultural dupes, but rather as individuals able to resist performative ideals of the virtuous bio-citizen. Our analysis of the girls' critique resonates with Foucault's belief that discourse can be created, negotiated and resisted.

The girls also critically reflected upon the potential use of digital health technologies in their PE lessons. They frequently emphasised that they valued the holistic, social interactive nature of PE, as this was often absent in their other classes at school. The girls agreed that the repetitive nature of workout based apps would not be advantageous within the PE curriculum, nor would these technologies appeal to the less athletic pupils:

> Grace: I think part of the fact why taking part in sport and fitness is fun is because you have other people around you. I know a lot of my sports are based around making friendships and a lot of people get that out of going to fitness classes, you make new friends and I think that's part of what makes it fun. Whereas with the apps it's quite individual, it's not about social interaction.
>
> Zoe: … pupils would get very bored very quickly and it wouldn't appeal to the less athletic people.

The girls all agreed that the social and community aspects of sport, such as communication and team-work, were more important than digital devices. Rather than focusing entirely upon their own engagement with apps, the girls also reflected upon other individuals whom they perceived to need motivation to engage in sport. By juxtaposing their own perspectives of apps with other 'less athletic' individuals, the participants reinforced their own embodied identities as motivated and 'sporty'. It is, therefore, important to reflect upon this presentation of the self and the girls' status as Sports Leaders in the school; the girls each held the embodied sense of self as a confident and 'sporty' role model, and associated socialising and enjoyment with their PE lessons. The girls were embedded in sporting cultures and held the social privilege to engage with health and fitness apps, yet at the same time they confidently rejected these technologies for removing the social aspects of sport they valued. If we had conducted focus groups with a group of adolescent girls who were disengaged from sport, their responses to the social environment of PE would have likely been different. This is particularly salient, as previous research exploring adolescent girls' embodied and social experiences within PE lessons has illustrated that girls often feel self-conscious, unhappy and uncomfortable within PE classes (Knowles, Niven, & Fawkner, 2014).

Digital health technologies have been considered as individual, motivational devices to encourage young people to participate in sport and physical activity (Lupton, 2013). Yet this group of female adolescents critiqued the isolating focus on toning one's body emphasised by devices, as this would be detrimental to their long-term engagement in sport. This final section has illustrated the girls' adoption of alternative discourses to critique health and fitness apps for the loss of sociality, unrealistic classifications of 'normal' BMI and assumption that apps can help individuals achieve an 'ideal body'. As Millie claimed, 'you can't really define a normal ideal weight, obviously people have different perceptions of what it is'.

Conclusion

This paper is a response to the need for in-depth analysis of individuals' 'subjectivities and embodiment in the world of m-health' (Lupton, 2012, p. 241). When faced with the task of examining the degree to which health and fitness apps are about health or about controlling the body, this research has engaged with the nuances, resistances and contradictions around the multiple meanings of health within our digital society. The findings reveal it is imperative to move not only beyond considerations of adolescents as docile, cultural dupes, but also beyond the totalising effects of pedagogical, digital spaces. Indeed, the participant-led innovative and interactive tasks were central to providing the girls with opportunities to express critical understandings of unrealistic ideals of slenderness as representative of health.

Guided by Foucault's conceptualisations of discourse, bio-power and technologies of the self, we have examined the adolescent girls' negotiation of the ambiguities surrounding neoliberal health discourses that manifested affectively and relationally through the self-monitoring technologies. At times during the focus group meetings, the girls reinforced restrictive understandings of health as a responsibility of individuals. They illustrated how, through promoting the imperative to be accountable for one's health, health and fitness apps could encourage citizens to be more healthy and simultaneously help combat the so-called 'obesity epidemic'. Moreover, the girls' engagement in social media alongside health and fitness apps resonated with the online social media trend of 'fitspiration', whereby individuals are inspired to engage in an active lifestyle through sharing a commitment to functional exercise and healthy food (Tiggemann & Zaccardo, 2015). The girls' narratives around the 'before and after' image as being a fitness motivation emphasised how social and popular media spaces can promote narrow ideals of slenderness and, when used alongside health and fitness apps, reinforce the 'corporeal' responsibility upon adolescents to direct surveillance onto their own bodies.

It is important to acknowledge that these English adolescent girls also understood critical and holistic notions of health, whilst emphasised the potential negative implications of engaging with health and fitness apps. They were particularly critical that health and fitness apps, similar to popular media, promoted a slim, 'ideal' body that is unobtainable for most. The girls were further critical of apps and other digital gaming technologies for using limiting measures of BMI to label a 'normal' body. According to Lupton (2013), instead of empowering individuals, digital health technologies increase the visibility of one's health, which can be perceived as a burden and create greater anxiety amongst individuals. Moreover, the girls articulated that digital technologies and social media disregard how individuals feel and should instead accept a diversity of body sizes as representative of health.

The girls all agreed that social interaction through physical activity and sport was important to them. They simultaneously critiqued the individual nature of apps for isolating individuals and removing the holistic characteristics of healthy lifestyles they valued; being active in a fun environment, socialising and competing with friends. This appreciation for the community nature of sport engagement is highly significant. As digitised health promotion is increasingly considered to combat physical activity drop-out rates for young individuals (Lupton, 2013), it is imperative to acknowledge the subjectivities of adolescents and what is valued within their everyday lives. Therefore, it is important to acknowledge how this group of adolescent girls perceived health and fitness apps would isolate adolescents and could be detrimental to their long-term engagement in physical activity. Future in-depth research around digitised health promotion may involve examining both pupils' and PE teachers' perspectives of the implications of technology upon traditional social interaction within PE.

Throughout this paper, we have emphasised it is important to consider the influence of the girls' status as Sports Leaders, embedded within a sporting culture at a relatively privileged grammar school in the UK. While the girls themselves did not reflect upon their class or their engagement in health and fitness apps in 'classed' terms, we have engaged in the nuances of dominant health imperatives within the girls' particular social worlds. This reflexive engagement is central to emphasising that the perspectives within this study were not representative of all adolescent girls. We also need to be mindful that adolescent boys can be equally vulnerable to pressures to conform to societal bodily values as their female peers (Grogan, 2007). Further research needs to engage with the perspectives of both male and female adolescents from different social, economic and cultural backgrounds, in order to facilitate a better understanding of the role of digital health technologies in the lives of various young individuals.

Finally, it is necessary that health promotion practitioners and academics confront the consequences of these developments, particularly as today's young digital natives are increasingly interacting with self-monitoring technologies (Millington, 2009). We have raised the possibilities for thinking about how, when given the opportunity through creative tasks, adolescents can engage in critical conversations about health and the body portrayed by health and fitness apps and wider media. Azzarito (2010) highlights that 'Schools might function as critical sites of resistance to and transformation of contemporary dominant discourses about the female body' (p. 270). Furthermore, it is imperative that public health, schools and future social scientific research considers individuals' affective and subjective responses to digital health technologies that are highly significant to their level of sustained engagement in physical activity. This study has illustrated how digital health technologies can provide possibilities for young individuals' health promotion, yet careful considerations for how the concept of 'health' is represented are necessary.

References

Azzarito, L. (2010). Future girls, transcendent femininities and new pedagogies: Toward girls' hybrid bodies? *Sport, Education and Society, 15,* 261–275. doi:10.1080/13573322.2010.493307

Beausoleil, N. (2009). An impossible task?: Preventing disordered eating in the context of the current obesity panic. In J. Wright & V. Harwood (Eds.), *Governing bodies: Biopolitics and the 'obesity epidemic'* (pp. 93–107). London: Routledge.

Cummiskey, M. (2011). There's an app for that: Smartphone use in health and physical education. *The Journal of Physical Education, Recreation & Dance, 82,* 24–30. doi:10.1080/07303084.2011.10598672

Evans, J., Rich, E., & Holroyd, R. (2004). Disordered eating and disordered schooling: What schools do to middle class girls. *British Journal of Sociology of Education, 25,* 123–142. doi:10.1080/0142569042000205154

Foucault, M. (1978). *The history of sexuality, volume 1: An introduction.* (R. Hurley, Trans.). New York, NY: Random House.

Foucault, M. (1984). The politics of health in the eighteenth century. In P. Rabinow (Ed.), *The Foucault reader* (pp. 273–289). New York, NY: Pantheon Books.

Foucault, M. (1988). *Discipline and punish: The birth of the prison.* London: Penguin.

Gard, M., & Wright, J. (2001). Obesity discourses and physical education in a risk society. *Studies in Philosophy and Education, 20,* 535–549. doi:10.1023/A:1012238617836

Grogan, S. (2007). *Body image: Understanding body dissatisfaction in men, women and children.* New York, NY: Routledge.

Guillemin, M., & Gillam, L. (2004). Ethics, reflexivity, and 'ethically important moments' in research. *Qualitative Inquiry, 10*, 261–280. doi:10.1177/1077800403262360

Halse, C., Honey, A., & Boughtwood, D. (2007). The paradox of virtue: (Re)thinking deviance, anorexia and schooling. *Gender and Education, 19*, 219–235. doi:10.1080/09540250601166068

Harwood, V. (2009). Theorizing biopedagogies. In J. Wright & V. Harwood (Eds.), *Governing bodies: Biopolitics and the 'obesity epidemic'* (pp. 15–30). London: Routledge.

Jutel, A. (2006). The emergence of overweight as a disease entity: Measuring up normality. *Social Science and Medicine, 63*, 2268–2276. doi:10.1016/j.socscimed.2006.05.028

Knowles, A. M., Niven, A., & Fawkner, S. (2014). 'Once upon a time I used to be active'. Adopting a narrative approach to understanding physical activity behaviour in adolescent girls. *Qualitative Research in Sport, Exercise and Health, 6*, 62–76. doi:10.1080/2159676X.2013.766816

Lupton, D. (1995). *The imperative of health: Public health and the regulated body.* London: Sage.

Lupton, D. (2012). M-Health and health promotion: The digital cyborg and surveillance society. *Social Theory & Health, 10*, 229–244. doi:10.1057/sth.2012.6

Lupton, D. (2013). Quantifying the body: Monitoring and measuring health in the age of mHealth technologies. *Critical Public Health, 23*, 393–403. doi:10.1080/09581596.2013.794931

Lupton, D. (2015). Health promotion in the digital era: A critical commentary. *Health Promotion International, 30*(1), 174–183. doi:10.1093/heapro/dau091

Markula, P. (2001). Firm but shapely, fit but sexy, strong but thin: The postmodern aerobicizing female bodies. In A. Yiannakis & M. J. Melnick (Eds.), *Contemporary issues in sociology of sport* (pp. 237–360). Champaign, IL: Human Kinetics.

Markula, P. (2004). 'Tuning into oneself:' Foucault's technologies of the self and mindful fitness. *Sociology of Sport Journal, 21*, 302–321. Retrieved from http://web.b.ebscohost.com/ehost/pdfviewer/pdfviewer?sid=03c8355c-bddc-497c-b64d-46f043c5c8ce%40sessionmgr120&vid=2&hid=128

Markula, P., & Silk, M. (2011). *Qualitative research for physical culture.* New York, NY: Palgrave Macmillan.

Marwick, A. E. (2012). The public domain: Social surveillance in everyday life. *Surveillance & Society, 9*, 378–393. Retrieved from http://library.queensu.ca/ojs/index.php/surveillance-and-society/article/view/pub_dom

McEvilly, N., Atencio, M., Verheul, M., & Jess, M. (2013). Understanding the rationale for pre-school physical education: Implications for practitioners' and children's embodied practices and subjectivity formation. *Sport, Education and Society, 18*, 731–748. doi:10.1080/13573322.2011.606807

Millington, B. (2009). Wii has never been modern: 'Active video' games and the 'conduct of conduct'. *New Media & Society, 11*, 621–640. doi:10.1177/1461444809102966

Nichols, R., Davis, K. L., McCord, T., Schmidt, D., & Slezak, A. M. (2009). The use of heart rate monitors in physical education. *Strategies: A Journal for Physical and Sport Educators, 22*, 19–23. doi:10.1080/08924562.2009.10590845

Ofcom. (2011, August 4). A nation addicted to smartphones. *Ofcom report.* Retrieved from http://media.ofcom.org.uk/news/2011/a-nation-addicted-to-smartphones/

Ohman, M., Almqvist, J., Meckbach, J., & Quennerstedt, M. (2014). Competing for ideal bodies: A study of exergames used as teaching aids in schools. *Critical Public Health, 24*, 196–209. doi:10.1080/09581596.2013.872771

Quraishi, S., & Quraishi, H. (2012). Freedom HIV/AIDS: Mobile phone games for health communication and behaviour change. In J. Donner & P. Mechael (Eds.), *mHealth in Practice: Mobile technology for health promotion in the developing world* (pp. 146–161). London: Bloomsbury.

Rabinow, P. (1991). *The Foucault reader.* London: Penguin.

Rich, E. (2011a). 'I see her being obesed!': Public pedagogy, reality media and the obesity crisis. *Health, 15*, 3–21. doi:10.1177/1363459309358127

Rich, E. (2011b). Exploring the relationship between pedagogy and physical cultural studies: The case of new health imperatives in schools. *Sociology of Sport Journal, 28*(1), 64–84. Retrieved from http://journals.humankinetics.com/ssj-back-issues/ssj-volume-28-issue-1-march/exploring-the-relationship-between-pedagogy-and-physical-cultural-studies-the-case-of-new-health-imperatives-in-schools

Rich, E., & Miah, A. (2009). Prosthetic surveillance: The medical governance of healthy bodies in cyberspace. *Surveillance & Society, 6,* 163–177. Retrieved from http://queens.scholarsportal.info/ojs/index.php/surveillance-and-society/article/view/3256

Rich, E., & Miah, A. (2014). Understanding digital health as public pedagogy: A critical framework. *Societies, 4,* 296–315. doi:103390/soc4020296

Sparkes, A. C., & Smith, B. (2014). *Qualitative research methods in sport, exercise and health: From process to product.* Oxon: Routledge.

Sport England. (2015). *Active design. Planning for health and wellbeing through sport and physical activity.* Retrieved from https://www.sportengland.org/media/1036460/spe003-active-design-published-october-2015-high-quality-for-web-2.pdf

Tiggemann, M., & Zaccardo, M. (2015). 'Exercise to be fit, not skinny': The effect of fitspiration imagery on women's body image. *Body Image, 15,* 61–67. doi:10.1016/j.bodyim.2015.06.003

Vander Schee, C. J., & Boyles, D. (2010). 'Exergaming', corporate interests and the crisis discourse of childhood obesity. *Sport, Education and Society, 15,* 169–185. doi:10.1080/135733210036 83828

Wachs, F. L., & Chase, L. F. (2013). Explaining the failure of an obesity intervention: Combining Bourdieu's symbolic violence and the Foucault's microphysics of power to reconsider state interventions. *Sociology of Sport Journal, 30,* 111–131. Retrieved from http://www.fitnessforlife.org/AcuCustom/Sitename/Documents/DocumentItem/01_wachs_SSJ_20120047_111-131-ej.pdf

Wright, J., & Halse, C. (2014). The healthy child citizen: Biopedagogies and web-based health promotion. *British Journal of Sociology of Education, 35,* 837–855. doi:10.1080/01425692.2013.800446

Wright, J., O'Flynn, G., & Macdonald, D. (2006). Being fit and looking healthy: Young women's and men's constructions of health and fitness. *Sex Roles, 54,* 707–716. doi:10.1007/s11199-006-9036-9

Index

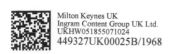

9 780367 321864